The Mother's Book of HOME MEDICAL TESTS for Infants & Children

THE MOTHER'S BOOK OF HOME MEDICAL TESTS FOR INFANTS & CHILDREN

Herbert Haessler, M.D.
author of *Medical Tests You Can Do Yourself*

and Raymond Harris

CB

CONTEMPORARY BOOKS

Library of Congress Cataloging-in-Publication Data

Haessler, Herbert.
    The mother's book of home medical tests for infants & children :
more than 200 at-home examinations and observations / Herbert
Haessler and Raymond Harris.
        p.   cm.
    ISBN 0-8092-3037-2
    1. Infants—Health and hygiene.   2. Infants—Medical
examinations. 3. Infants—Diseases—Diagnosis.   4. Physical
diagnosis—Popular works.   5. Pediatrics—Popular works.   I. Harris,
Raymond Herman.   II. Title.
RJ61.H1483   1998
618.92—dc21   98-10365
                                                    CIP

Cover design by Nick Panos
Cover illustration by Joyce Stiglich
Interior drawings by Brunelle Graphics
Interior design by City Desktop Productions

Published by Contemporary Books
A division of NTC/Contemporary Publishing Group, Inc.
4255 West Touhy Avenue, Lincolnwood (Chicago), Illinois 60646-1975 U.S.A.
Printed in the United States of America
International Standard Book Number: 0-8092-3037-2
18   17   16   15   14   13   12   11   10   9   8   7   6   5   4   3   2

This book is dedicated to the babies we have known, who have become adults in a remarkably short space of time and are now parents themselves; to Julie and Heidi Scanlon; Olivia, Nicholas, and Thomas Harris; and to those who are still to come.

Special thanks are due to Diane Haessler, B.S., R.N.P., whose extensive experience in pediatric nursing and her critical eye for detail have contributed immeasurably to this book.

CONTENTS

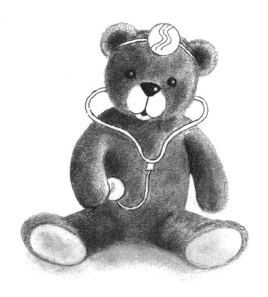

INTRODUCTION

WHY PARENTS SHOULD EXAMINE THEIR BABY AT HOME

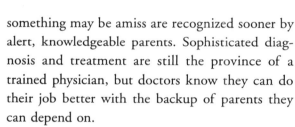

You know from experience that the more familiar you are with something you have to do, the more confident you are doing it. This is especially true when it comes to caring for new babies and young children. The more you know about little bodies, how they function, how they are supposed to look when they are well and happy, and how they might look and act when they are not, the more confident you will be in fulfilling your function as principal guardian of your baby's healthy growth and development.

Confidence in dealing with new babies and young children comes from two sources— experience and knowledge. Experience begins the first time you hold your baby. And the best way to begin to acquire knowledge about babies is to take a good look at your own in an organized way. This means a careful examination of baby's body and baby's responses as a newborn and at regular intervals afterward.

Realizing their time limitations, doctors now emphasize that the primary responsibility for monitoring the health and normal development of children rests with parents. Early warnings that something may be amiss are recognized sooner by alert, knowledgeable parents. Sophisticated diagnosis and treatment are still the province of a trained physician, but doctors know they can do their job better with the backup of parents they can depend on.

It is only good sense for parents to know their baby intimately, to know their baby's normals so that they can tell when something is wrong. It makes sense, too, that once parents recognize a problem, they should know what they can handle, what should be seen by a doctor, and what constitutes a medical emergency.

In the following pages, you will find a wealth of information about examining and caring for your baby. There is nothing difficult about it, and it requires nothing in the way of complicated instruments or specialized knowledge. And getting to know your baby as intimately as we recommend is a fascinating exercise in parenthood that will be one of your most rewarding experiences.

Here, summarized in question-and-answer form, are some basic things you will probably want to know about home examination.

Why Should I Examine My Baby?

Why not examine your baby? He is yours, after all, and he'll probably enjoy the attention. (Throughout this book we refer to babies alternately as either "he" or "she" to avoid the cumbersome expression "he or she." We love girls and boys equally.) You, in turn, will learn a great deal about your baby, and you will be in a much better position to judge when things are going well and when they are not. No one sees your baby on a day-to-day basis as you do. So no one, including the doctor, is better qualified than you are to watch over your baby's health and to monitor your baby's growth and development.

Shouldn't a Baby Be Seen Regularly by a Doctor?

Definitely yes! It is generally recommended that new babies see a doctor fairly often during the first year and then less frequently after that. A doctor should become familiar with your baby, assure you that she's healthy, answer all your questions, set up a feeding and nutrition schedule, and supervise an inoculation program (this is very important). The doctor will want a history of your baby, her family background, the story of your pregnancy and delivery, and the doctor will want to track the baby's growth.

If the Doctor Does All That, What Do I Have to Do?

Parents should know everything the doctor knows about their baby and many other things besides. The doctor can't possibly know your baby and your baby's body as well as you do. The doctor sees the baby once a month, and that's only in the early

months. You see your baby every day and will continue to do so after visits to the doctor dwindle to every three months and then to once a year.

Doctors must work with averages that are based on seeing many babies. You work with one individual. It is important, for example, to know what is a normal temperature for your baby. All "normals" aren't the same. And the "normal" a baby registers on one visit to the doctor may not represent his true normal at all. A normal temperature is determined by checking the baby's temperature at different times during the day.

Though under the best circumstances a doctor tracks a baby's growth regularly during the first year, it is important for you to have your own growth records of your baby that are tracked through puberty. People move and change doctors frequently, and records tend to get scattered if they are not transferred with each move or each change in health care.

It is important that you know your baby's symptoms of being well. This means knowing all of your baby and all of her body systems. If you don't know what all the normals look like in your baby, it is hard to determine—or even notice—when something is wrong that calls for a doctor's attention.

Some things simply serve to reassure parents. Does the baby hear? Are his eyes all right? Is he developing normally, and how do you know except that the doctor (whom you see infrequently) says so?

Can a Mother or Father Do All These Things?

Yes. The largest part of a physical examination of a baby (or of yourself, for that matter) consists of very simple things: measurements, taking temperature and pulse, listening to the heart (easy), checking blood pressure (extremely important for yourself, too), looking in the mouth and ears, and a number of other things that are just as uncomplicated and nontechnical.

What you look for are normal conditions. You can only recognize normal conditions if you are used to examining your baby regularly when she is well. When a deviation from normal appears, you want to know it and call it to the attention of the doctor. Most problems with babies, in fact, are first noticed by parents and then formally diagnosed by a doctor.

A most important part of a medical examination is the questioning part. This is the medical history, and it has been shown in studies that this part of the examination is so important that between 80 percent and 85 percent of all doctors' diagnoses of illness (or wellness) can be made on the basis of the history alone. The tests and examinations a doctor does are used largely to confirm suspicions and to better define problems.

A medical history begins with things as elementary as age, and it progresses through family background, when you first notice a particular difficulty, how the problem manifests itself, and what you have been doing about it. The more accurate the information that you are able to provide the doctor, the better job she can do in diagnosing and treating whatever the problem is.

As a practiced baby observer and examiner, you will have all your facts and records available in great detail; you will be able to talk with the doctor in an intelligent and informed manner, and the doctor will be able to talk to you in the same way.

Here are some of the things you can do better than a doctor:

- Establish your baby's normal ranges for temperature, pulse and heart rate, blood pressure, and respiration.

- Observe early signs of vision problems. Often a child's first vision screening isn't given until he starts school. This is too late to catch and correct some defects that a parent can find easily in the early years when correction is still possible.

- Track growth in terms of height, weight, head, and chest circumferences. Most doctors track this for you if the doctor sees a baby regularly during the first six months, but this stops when a doctor stops seeing a child regularly, even though it is important to continue the tracking right up to puberty.

- Spot development of skeletal defects. Most of the time, it is up to the parents to spot such defects in their early stages when they are most correctible. There are simple home tests for this.

- Keep a health history and health records. Parents can keep better records than a doctor can. A child's records often become scattered among many different doctors. It's easier for parents to keep complete family health records in one place for instant retrieval when they are needed.

A cloud of mystery sometimes seems to hang over the simplest (and most important) medical tests. Fortunately, there are signs that the cloud is dissipating. With the popularity of jogging and other exercise programs, millions of people have learned how to check vital life signs—the pulse, for example. The American Heart Association is responsible for getting people to check their own blood pressure. Breast self-examination has become universally recommended. And now there are do-it-yourself pregnancy tests and many other home tests on the shelf in your drugstore.

One barrier after another is falling as the medical profession and public have come to realize that there is much benefit to be gained when people keep track of how their body systems work. Throughout this book, you will find hundreds of tests, procedures, and observations that you can do for your baby. Many are valuable for adults, too. Most require no special equipment, while a few call for common medical tools—a thermometer, a stethoscope (anybody can use one), a blood pressure cuff, and so on.

Can I Hurt My Baby by Performing These Tests?

Absolutely not. As fragile as they look, babies are remarkably tough little critters who love to be handled. You want to be gentle, of course, but firm and confident in your approach. If you do this with medical testing, there is no more danger to your baby than there is in giving a bath, lifting her in and out of bed, or changing a diaper.

When a baby has been healthy and develops a common problem—a cold, earache, diarrhea—there are some perfectly safe and sensible things you can do to make him more comfortable and sometimes resolve the problem on your own.

What Do Doctors Think of All This?

Your doctor won't be a bit jealous that you have learned to do some of the things he can do. Modern physicians welcome the informed cooperation of intelligent parents. The most modern professionals will insist on your full cooperation as the only one who, in the final analysis, can do the things that are most necessary to maintain the health of your family.

But physicians don't appreciate parents who take it upon themselves to play doctor, whole hog, making positive diagnoses and prescribing treatment when it is obvious that a professional should be seen. Whenever there is a deviation from what you know is normal for your baby, the time has arrived to consult with your partner, the doctor. You needn't be embarrassed to tell her what you suspect is wrong as a result of your testing and observations; doctors want to know this. You may discuss and even question the doctor's findings if there is some question in your mind. But final diagnosis and treatment is properly the province of the other half of your team. If you disagree with your doctor's findings and prescribed treatment (this is permissible), discuss it. If you can't reach a solution, then it's time to find a new partner. At times of disagreement in a doctor–patient relationship, it's not at all unthinkable that a parent may be right and a doctor may be wrong. It happens.

Haven't Mothers and Fathers Always Looked After Their Babies' Health?

Yes, but many errors have been made for want of knowledge about babies that can be avoided when organized information is put to work in support of traditional care and your intuitive feeling for what's right.

Higher levels of general education among parents, and enlightened attitudes among doctors, are rapidly changing the way health care is administered. More responsibility is being placed on individuals to look after themselves and their children. The enthusiasm for bringing families into the health care process is growing so fast, in fact, that this is where the next great leap forward will come in reducing illness and extending life, rather than from any new medicines or technologies. And it is appropriate that the process that can lead to a longer, healthier life begins with the newborn and the very young child.

We hope this book will encourage you to learn more about your baby and to participate in over-seeing your baby's health. We hope, too, that it will make you more knowledgeable, more observant, and more confident in dealing with your baby and better equipped to make the best use of whatever professional health care facilities are available in your community.

THE MOTHER'S BOOK OF

HOME MEDICAL TESTS

FOR INFANTS & CHILDREN

CHAPTER 1

THE FIRST EXAMINATION OF YOUR NEWBORN BABY

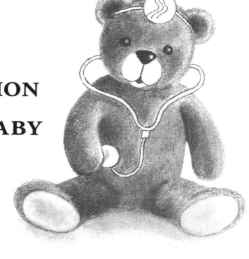

A newborn baby has a helpless, fragile appearance. The head looks too large, the legs too short. He seems barrel-chested and flat-bottomed. He is covered all over with a whitish, greasy material, streaked with blood from the delivery, and he sports a shimmering, translucent cord at the center of his slightly potty abdomen. There's no getting away from it—a newborn baby can be odd looking. At the same time, he is also tremendously appealing, and the first glimpse of their newborn seldom fails to inspire intense feelings of love and protectiveness in parents. At the back of their minds, however, another feeling emerges—one of apprehension. From the moment of birth, parents want to know, "Is our baby all right?"

Parents are eager to examine their baby to be sure that she is, indeed, all right. But after you've counted the fingers and the toes, what more can parents tell? Quite a bit, actually. Most of the tests, measurements, and observations that the doctor uses to check a newborn baby can be duplicated at home by parents.

The Apgar Test

The first test your baby ever takes is administered one minute after birth, and the test is given again five minutes after birth. Called the Apgar Test, it measures a newborn's well-being. Coming as it does immediately after delivery, this is one test you will have to leave up to the doctor or other professional birth attendants. But you should ask the doctor how your baby scored on the Apgar Test. Make a note of the results to enter in your baby's personal health record, which we will discuss in Chapter 17, "How to Create a Medical History and Health Record for Your Baby."

There are five parts to the Apgar Test, and each part receives a score of either 0, 1, or 2 points. Therefore, 10 is a perfect score. The items are scored as follows:

HEART RATE. Using a stethoscope to listen to the heart, the doctor counts the number of beats per minute and assigns a score of 0 (heartbeat absent), 1 (less than 100 beats per minute), or 2 (greater than 100 beats per minute).

1

RESPIRATORY EFFORT. Observing the infant's breathing, the doctor gives 0 if breathing is absent, 1 point if it is slow or irregular, and 2 points if breathing is good or if the baby is crying.

MUSCLE TONE. The baby receives 0 if muscles are limp, 1 if some movement is apparent, and 2 for active motion of the arms and legs.

COLOR. An infant that is bluish or pale all over receives a score of 0. If body color is good but the color of the arms and legs is poor (bluish or gray-white), a score of 1 is given. Good color of both the body and the extremities merits a score of 2.

RESPONSE TO SUCTION TUBE IN NOSTRIL. No response results in a score of 0; a facial grimace rates 1, and a cough or sneeze receives 2 points.

The second test score—the five-minute score—is the more useful in terms of predicting how well the baby is likely to fare in the future. A baby in good condition is likely to achieve an Apgar score of 7 to 10 points. Infants with scores of 4 to 6 are considered to be in guarded condition and will be watched intensively for the first few days of life. Scores of 3 or less reflect a critical state requiring emergency measures to save the infant's life.

The Three Stages of Birth Recovery

Mother and baby are soon introduced to each other and the baby is tagged, weighed, footprinted, and bathed. The baby now passes through three stages of birth recovery. You will want to observe this period of recovery or adjustment to its new life as part of your first examination.

STAGE ONE. The first stage of birth recovery begins with an infant's first breath and lasts for approximately thirty to sixty minutes. During this first period, the newborn is wide-eyed and alert. He will likely flex his muscles, make facial grimaces, and cry.

STAGE TWO. Within an hour after birth, the first flurry of activity subsides. The heart rate decreases, the respiratory rate decreases, the general muscle tone and level of activity wind down, and the infant sleeps for three to four hours.

STAGE THREE. A second period of activity begins about the fourth or fifth hour after birth. The baby awakens and begins to size up his new environment, moves his head from side to side, opens and closes his eyes, twitches his nostrils, purses his lips, sticks out his tongue, brandishes his arms and legs, and so on. He may pass the contents of his bowels into his diaper and give a loud cry of hunger.

If all is well, baby is usually given to the mother to hold and put to the breast shortly after the immediate birth procedures have been attended to. Both mother and baby enjoy the experience, and the stimulation of the suckling helps the uterus to contract. Newborn babies think their mothers look pretty good. First-time mothers, on the other hand, are frequently dismayed by various aspects of their newborn's appearance. Too often they are unprepared for the "stork bites," the puffy eyes, or any of a number of other common, and usually temporary, characteristics of the newborn. Knowing what to expect can forestall a gulp of dismay.

Examining Your Newborn's Head

New parents are concerned about their newborn's head. For one thing, it looks abnormally large, taking up fully a quarter of a newborn's total body length—about twice the proportion of an adult's head. Its shape may appear somewhat elongated because the head may be slightly molded as it passes through the birth canal. The effect is only temporary, however, and the head returns to its normal shape within a few weeks.

Another mark often left by the delivery process is a soft, spongy area on the top of the head caused by the pressure against the baby's head during birth. Called *caput succedaneum*, or simply caput, this soft swelling is actually a very minor injury to the soft tissue on the top of the head and generally heals within a week.

A somewhat harder swelling over the top of the head occasionally results from bleeding under the surface of one of the soft bones of the skull. This condition is limited to one side of the head. This harder swelling may have a soft spot in the center, which is of no significance and is simply a reflection of how the bleeding has distributed itself. These swellings caused by bleeding take somewhat longer to resolve than the softer swelling of the caput, and, though worrisome to parents, they rarely have any permanent significance.

Forceps are rarely used today, but if the doctor does have to use forceps to assist the baby's progress through the birth canal, you may notice a few slight dents over the face and head. Forceps are something like the kitchen tool you use to lift hot vegetables out of a pot but with carefully smoothed and rounded edges. The dents that you see are left by the rims of the forceps. These marks are usually just a bit red, although they may occasionally develop into black-and-blue marks. They'll disappear within a few days.

You will also be able to detect areas in your baby's skull where the bones have not yet fused. These gaps, known as the *fontanels*, or simply soft spots, are covered with a tough membrane that will eventually ossify and become bone. The membrane is quite good protection in the meantime, and there is no need to be unduly concerned about touching the head when washing or caressing it.

Locating the Fontanels

There are two fontanels of practical importance in a baby's skull. Both are located on the midline—one toward the back of the skull (the posterior fontanel) and one on the top (the anterior fontanel). There are also two soft spots on each side of the head where the bones of the skull have not fused at birth. These are difficult to detect, however, and close up relatively early, within a month or so after birth.

The posterior fontanel, located on the midline toward the base of the skull, is also small—about the size of the tip of your finger. It closes within a few months after birth. The largest of the soft spots is the anterior fontanel, located on the midline at the top of the head. This diamond-shaped area may be as large as two inches across and will not be completely filled in with bone until the middle of the baby's second year.

The anterior fontanel at the top of the head tends to bulge slightly when the baby lies down or cries, and to sink in a bit when the baby is sitting up quietly. However, **a bulging anterior fontanel in**

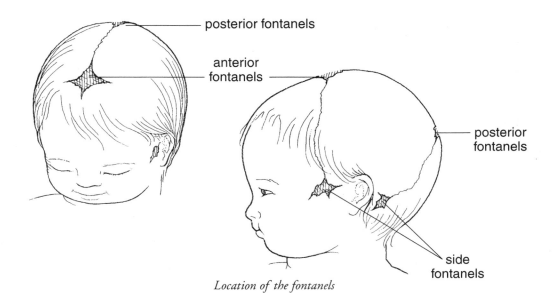

Location of the fontanels

a quiet, apparently sick baby is an ominous sign and should be treated as a medical emergency.

In addition to these soft spots, the lines along which the bones of the skull meet on the top of the head can also be felt in some newborns. These joinings are called sutures, and sometimes open up just a little during the birth process; occasionally the pressure may be such that one bone temporarily rides up on another. If this has happened, the overriding bones will soon slip back into their normal position.

Measuring Head Circumference

As large as it seems at birth, the head continues to grow at a fairly rapid pace. Head circumference, in fact, is a particularly important measurement of an infant's growth and development, especially in the first six months of life.

To measure your newborn's head circumference, place a tape measure around the baby's head, crossing the forehead just above the eyes and going back just above the ears. Several measurements should be taken at slightly different locations and the largest value used. Normal head size of a newborn ranges from about 33 to 37 centimeters (13 to 14½ inches).

Measuring and tracking your newborn's head circumference on a regular basis can help you to detect a relatively uncommon but potentially life-threatening condition called *hydrocephalus*, which is an abnormal accumulation of fluid within the skull and is characterized by enlargement of the head. Bulging fontanels are one of the earliest signs. If not treated promptly, brain damage and possibly death can result. By plotting your baby's head circumference on the appropriate growth chart as described in Chapter 14, you can compare her measurements with average head circumferences from birth through thirty-six months. If your baby's head circumference seems abnormally large or is increasing more rapidly than it should according to the chart, check with the doctor promptly. And if suture lines of the skull seem to be widening, this should also be brought to the attention of the doctor.

It's hard to examine your newborn's head without remarking on the presence—or absence—of hair. Some babies are born with a considerable amount of hair on the head, whereas others have little, if any. The amount of hair at the time of birth has no significance. Gradually over the first year of life, a full head of hair will develop.

Examining Your Newborn's Eyes and Vision

By the time your infant has passed through the three stages of the birth recovery and is ready for its first feeding, you should be able to observe the pupillary response and perform a rudimentary vision check.

Observing the Pupillary Response

If you shine a flashlight into the baby's eyes when he is awake and alert (just a quick on and off), you'll notice that the pupil—the black area in the center of the eye—constricts slightly as a result of the light stimulus. This is the pupillary response. If you can't catch a pupillary response, a tight blink and a frown tells you that the baby is aware of the light.

Checking Vision

Though you cannot determine how sharply your newborn sees, you can usually ascertain that vision is intact by observing her ability to follow a moving light or other stimulus.

Using your flashlight or a brightly colored ball, bring it within eight to twelve inches of baby's face and try to get the baby to follow the moving object

or to just turn her eyes a bit as it moves. Some newborns are better at this than others. A few will focus on a moving object and follow it over a considerable arc. Others may not follow the stimulus at all. The majority, however, will exhibit some response indicating that they see the stimulus.

You may have to try over and over again, but if you get just one positive response, you may assume that your baby's vision is intact. Keep in mind, too, that your baby may not be interested in performing for you at that moment, so a whole series of negative tests does not necessarily mean that your baby cannot see. It probably means that your baby does not feel like playing this game right now. Try again some other time.

Examining Your Newborn's Mouth

The mouth is the most active part of the newborn. Long before birth a fetus begins practicing mouth movements, so you'll find your newborn quite adept at pursing his lips, sticking out his tongue, swallowing, making interesting sounds, and, of course, crying. Two important reflexes can be observed here: the rooting reflex and the sucking reflex.

Eliciting the Rooting Reflex

To "root out" something means to search for it, and the rooting reflex is actually a newborn's search for the nipple—nourishment, in other words. Stroke the baby's cheek just to one side of the mouth. The newborn will respond by moving his head from side to side in search of the stimulus and may make a clumsy attempt to take the stroking finger into his mouth.

Observing the Sucking Reflex

Put the tip of your little finger into the baby's mouth. The newborn's lips will close on your finger, and he will commence sucking with considerable energy. (The sucking and rooting responses may be absent temporarily if the baby has just been fed.) Biting movements, rather than sucking movements, are abnormal responses and should be brought to the attention of the doctor.

You can examine the inside of your newborn's mouth by using a flashlight and the handle of a flat-handled spoon to gently hold down the baby's lower lip and tongue. You may see several small white spots along the gum margins. These are called *epithelial pearls*. They disappear within a short period of time and have no significance. On rare occasions, newborn babies have one or more soft front teeth. Your doctor may advise that these teeth be removed because of the possibility that one will be breathed into the lungs when the teeth fall out.

Examining Your Newborn's Skin

After the head, the newborn's skin receives a parent's closest scrutiny. Probably the most startling aspect of a newborn's skin is the whitish, greasy substance called vernix *caseosa*, covering the body at birth. The word *caseosa* means resembling cheese. This material is wiped off shortly after birth, but traces of it may be found in skin folds for a day or two.

Some newborns, particularly those born prematurely, are covered with very fine hair. Doctors refer to this as lanugo hair, and it disappears within a few days after birth. Infants who are born late—more than nine months gestation—often have noticeably dry skin, and there may be some crack-

ing and peeling. This is of little significance since perfectly normal skin is underneath.

Skin color can be affected by a number of common and usually passing conditions. For the first few hours after birth, the blood circulation near the surface of the body is increased, giving the infant an exaggerated color. This is particularly noticeable in light-skinned babies, but normal skin color soon becomes evident.

Often the hands and feet of newborns will have a bluish tinge, especially when they become even slightly cool. This condition is called peripheral cyanosis and has no particular significance other than that the baby is a bit chilly. However, a bluish color over the *entire* body is very significant. The infant is then often referred to as a "blue baby" and is likely to have a problem with its heart or lungs. A blue baby requires immediate medical attention.

Many infants develop some degree of yellow jaundice within the first few days after birth. Yellow jaundice is a general yellowish discoloration of the skin and the whites of the eyes. When severely jaundiced, the baby may have an almost orange appearance; more commonly, however, only a slight yellowing is apparent. If the condition is mild and slow in onset, it has very little significance. The slight discoloration disappears spontaneously after two or three days. More pronounced jaundice, however, particularly when it begins within the first day of life, is more serious and requires medical attention. The jaundiced baby is likely to be placed in a specially constructed incubator with a light array over the top, or in other similar devices. The baby's eyes are protected and the skin is continually exposed to the lights. Since bilirubin, the substance that causes jaundice, is destroyed by light when it passes through the surface of the skin, these light devices are an effective treatment for this condition.

An assortment of blemishes can affect the skin of newborns, and you should not be alarmed if your infant sports one of them. Most of them gradually disappear and none of them signify a life-threatening condition. You will find more detailed descriptions of birthmarks and other variations on normal skin in Chapter 2, "How to Examine Your Baby's Skin."

Examining the Abdomen and Umbilical Stump

The remnant of your newborn's old life support system—the umbilical cord—remains attached to the baby's abdomen for the first seven to ten days of life. The umbilical cord supplies the baby with nutrients from the mother. It also gets rid of metabolic wastes. If your doctor places your infant on your stomach immediately after delivery, as many do, you will be able to feel the blood pulsing through the umbilical cord before it is cut.

The cord's surface appears almost jelly-like, but it is far firmer than jelly. A careful inspection of the cut end of the cord will reveal that it contains three blood vessels—two arteries and one vein. The two arteries are heavy-walled tubes, whereas the vein, while somewhat larger in diameter, has a thinner wall.

The umbilical cord is often painted with an antiseptic solution to cut down the chances of infection of the umbilical stump. Over a period of about ten days, the umbilical cord dries, shrinks, and eventually falls off. During the drying period, it becomes hard and brown, much like a scab that forms on your skin after an injury. Like a scab, when it falls off it leaves a fresh pink area underneath it. Within a few days, this becomes the color of the surrounding skin, and the familiar navel or belly button remains.

Although the stump of the umbilical cord usually presents no problems, you should be aware of two conditions that may require a doctor's attention: an infection of the umbilical stump and an umbilical hernia.

Recognizing an Infection of the Umbilical Stump

Infection is indicated by a general reddening and perhaps swelling around the base of the cord. Infections in very young infants are not necessarily accompanied by fever. They are nonetheless serious, and anything more than a very slight pinkness around the base of the cord should be brought to the attention of your doctor promptly.

Identifying an Umbilical Hernia

A hernia is a portion of tissue or part of an organ that has protruded through a weakness or abnormal opening in the supporting walls that surround it. Small umbilical hernias are not uncommon in newborns. These can occur when incomplete central fusion of the abdominal muscles allows a piece of intestine to bulge through.

An umbilical hernia can be identified by an out-pouching in the area of the umbilicus. These hernias can be reduced by simple manual pressure, using your fingers to manipulate the contents of the hernia back into the abdomen. The hernia is likely to reoccur whenever the baby cries or strains. The vast majority of these umbilical hernias close spontaneously within the first year and need be no further cause for concern. Binders or pressure dressings are generally not recommended.

Examining the Genital Organs

Genital development in newborn boys varies widely. (Boys' genitals are discussed more fully in Chapter 11, "Checking on Baby's Bottom and Urinary System.") Most full-term boys have a well-developed scrotum (the pouch containing the testicles), with both testicles completely descended. Occasionally, however, one or both testicles are not in the scrotum, but are further up, in the abdomen where they originally formed. In such cases, the undescended testicle usually makes its appearance soon after birth.

The best time to observe your baby's scrotum is when he is in a warm bath. This is because the testicles are attached to muscles that draw them close to the groin on the slightest provocation—cold air, for example, or your cold, probing fingers. Try not to handle the scrotum at all when you look to see if the testicles are descended; the touch of your fingers alone may cause them to retract toward the body, giving you the mistaken impression that they are undescended. If a month or so has gone by, and one or both testicles seem not to have appeared in the scrotum, discuss it with your doctor. He will probably want to monitor the situation and perhaps take steps to correct it with a small surgical procedure by age three or four.

In newborn girls, the labia minora, or inner lips of the genitals, are very prominent at birth. (Girls' genitals are discussed more fully in Chapter 11.) In older infants, the labia majora, or outer lips, completely cover the smaller, inner lips as well as the vaginal opening and the urinary outlet, or urethra. You may notice a white, pink, or red mucous discharge containing some blood issuing from the vagina. This is a perfectly normal phe-

nomenon and is due to stimulation by the mother's hormones. These same hormones may also cause what appears to be some early breast development. There may be a definite fullness of the nipples, and sometimes colostrum, or "witch's milk," may be expressed from the nipple, in male as well as female infants. The vaginal discharge, the breast development, and the colostrum will gradually disappear within a few days after birth.

Hip Dysplasia

An important malformation involving the hip that may not be apparent at first glance is congenital hip dislocation. The hip joint is essentially a ball-and-socket arrangement in which the head of the femur, the upper leg bone, fits into the socket of the pelvis, or hip bones. In some infants, this socket does not develop properly and is too shallow to hold the ball of the femur in place. Consequently, when pressure is exerted at the joint, the ball of the femur tends to slip upward out of the socket, resulting in partial or complete dislocation of the hip.

Unless this deformity is detected in the first months of life, the condition may go unnoticed by parents until the child starts walking with a waddling gait. By this time, unfortunately, treatment is both difficult and unsatisfactory. The condition affects girls about five times as often as boys, and involves the left hip more frequently than the right.

How to Test for Hip Dysplasia

1. Place the baby on her back and bring both knees up to the belly and then—gently—out to the sides and downward. If either hip joint is improperly developed, you will feel resistance and may hear a snap, or click, as the upper leg

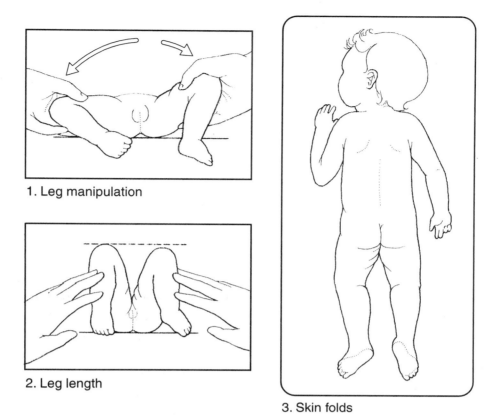

1. Leg manipulation

2. Leg length

3. Skin folds

Testing for hip dysplasia

bone slips out of the ball joint (be sure not to push too hard).

2. Another useful observation is leg length. With the baby lying on her back, bring both knees up and carefully study them from the front. If one knee seems lower than the other, this is another indication of possible hip malformation.

3. Finally, place the baby on a bed or table, face down, and observe the skin folds at the point where the upper legs join the buttocks. Several skin folds will be present at this point: there should be an equal number of folds on each

side. If hip dislocation is present, the affected side is likely to have an extra skin fold.

Congenital dislocation of the hip is not painful to the infant, but you must bring such a condition to the attention of your doctor promptly. Even a newborn can begin undergoing corrective treatment. (Treatment, however, should only be undertaken with the direction of a doctor.) The process consists of maintaining the upper legs in a full straddle position until the joint stabilizes. (Interestingly, it has been reported that in societies where mothers commonly carry their babies by having them straddle their back or hips, congenital hip dislocation is virtually unknown.)

For mild cases detected in the first weeks of life, the simple technique of double-diapering may be all that is needed to hold the legs at the proper angle. For older infants, there are casts, braces, pillow splints, and similar devices, all of which accomplish the correction. Treatment is usually completed within a matter of months.

Correction is vastly more involved for toddlers, however, and nearly impossible after the age of five or six. By this time, numerous muscles have permanently contracted and shortened to accommodate the displaced hip joint, and the bone itself has hardened. The result is a markedly shorter leg, spinal curvature, and a waddling walk.

Observing Respiration and Crying

One of the fundamental measures of a newborn's well-being is the respiratory rate—the number of times your baby breathes in and out in one minute. As noted earlier in the chapter, this measurement is one of the five parts that make up the Apgar Test given immediately after birth.

An infant's respiratory rate is significantly higher than your own. A normal adult rate varies between fourteen and twenty breaths per minute, whereas a newborn will breathe in and out about thirty times per minute. An easy way to check your baby's respiratory rate is to count the number of breaths in a fifteen-second interval and multiply by four.

As you count, observe the nature of your baby's breathing. The appearance of grunting respiration or a rattling sound when the baby takes a breath are both signs of trouble. In normal breath-

ing, the chest rises and falls and there is little deformity of the rib cage as the chest moves. Babies with respiratory problems, however, show some retraction of the ribs during breathing. The bones of a baby's chest are softer than the bones of an older child or an adult and tend to give more easily when breathing is not normal. Thus, when a baby with respiratory distress takes a deep breath, the central portion of the chest appears to sink in instead of moving outward. This finding would be associated with obvious breathing difficulty.

Crying is closely related to respiration simply because it takes a good set of lungs to produce a hearty cry. Healthy babies have a lusty cry that appears to be produced without a great deal of effort. Consistent high-pitched crying suggests trouble, as does a weak cry or a whining one. Crying patterns that differ substantially from the norm should be brought to the attention of your doctor.

Young babies do not cry without good reason. A crying baby is either hungry, startled, or uncomfortable (diaper may need changing), in pain, or perhaps in need of assurance or comforting. A baby who is "too good"—who never cries—actually may be an infant in trouble. Crying is a survival skill; it is the only method an infant has for communicating his needs. A baby who is apathetic and totally without complaints should be evaluated by a doctor.

Testing Reflexes and Fixed-Action Patterns

Newborn infants come equipped with a set of "fixed-action patterns," so called because they consist of a fixed series of movements that *all* normal infants exhibit. Some of these, like the sucking and rooting reflexes, are essential to the infant's survival. Others, like the grasp reflex described below, were probably more important early in human evolution but now seem to exist just to endear the newborn to the caregiver. Still other fixed-action patterns, such as the stepping reflex, seem to be precursors of skills the infant eventually acquires. Observation of these fixed-action patterns can be made in assessing the neurologic status of your newborn baby.

Observing the Traction Reflex

Place the baby on his back, grasp the hands and wrists, and gently pull the infant to a sitting position. The head at first lags, but then the baby makes an attempt to right his head; this should be almost completely accomplished when the baby has reached the sitting position. The test, of course, should be carried out slowly and gently, when the baby is fully awake and alert. The head will undoubtedly be unsteady; it's the attempt at control that is important. If no attempt at all is made to control the head, call this to a doctor's attention.

Observing the Grasp Reflex

The grasp reflex is elicited by stroking or merely touching the palm of the infant's hand with your finger, whereupon the infant will close her fingers over your own. This response lessens by the age of three to four months.

Eliciting the Righting Reflex

Lift your baby vertically from the table and he will bring his legs upward. Now touch the soles of the feet to a table and the baby will respond with the righting reflex—that is, his legs will extend, and his body and trunk will straighten up.

Observing the Stepping Reflex

After you have elicited the righting reflex described above, place the sole of one foot on the table until the baby steps with that leg; then place the other foot in contact with the table, and a similar reaction occurs. These alternate flexions of the leg resemble walking. The full-term infant will place the entire sole of the foot on the table, whereas the premature infant tends to walk on its toes.

Eliciting the Moro Reflex

Also called the startle reflex because of the manner in which the baby responds, this sequence of movements can be observed in infants up to eight or even twelve weeks old. The response can be elicited in almost any way that startles the infant. It is often elicited inadvertently when you bump into the crib with your knee or kick the crib with your foot. You can also elicit the Moro reflex by slapping the mattress of the crib briskly with your hand ten to twenty inches away from the baby's head.

The Moro response consists of a fixed set of movements: Simultaneously, the knees flex, the arms flail out, the fingers fan out; then, almost immediately, the arms are brought in close to the body, as if embracing something, and the fingers clench, thumb and index finger forming a "C" shape. There may be a slight tremor, then a return to normal movement. This startle reflex is accompanied by a vigorous cry.

An abnormal response is a notable lack of smoothness of the arm movement, such as jerkiness; a slow response is also abnormal, or a response that is markedly different on the baby's right and left sides.

Any test will depend on how the baby feels about cooperating at the moment, so don't give up after only one try. Three or four tries when the baby is in a good mood may be necessary to get a good result. Consistently abnormal responses, however, should be brought to the attention of the doctor.

Measuring Length and Weight

No examination of your newborn baby is complete without measuring three vital statistics: head circumference (described earlier), weight, and length. These measurements should be entered in your baby's health record. Length and weight measurements are taken in the delivery room immediately after birth, so you can get these first figures from your doctor or nurse.

Length

A baby's length is measured with the infant lying down, legs stretched out straight, and feet pointing more or less straight up. The measurement is taken from the soles of the feet at the heels to the top of the head. It is sometimes convenient to place the baby's feet against a flat vertical surface, like a wall, and then measure from the wall to the top of the baby's head. A normal full-term baby will usually be somewhere between 48 and 54 centimeters (19 to 21 inches) long. On the average, girls tend to be slightly smaller than boys at birth.

Weight

Weight at birth for a normal infant born after forty weeks' gestation (nine months' pregnancy) will be somewhere between 2500 and 3800 grams (5½ to 8½ pounds). This normal weight range should be adjusted slightly downward for babies born before forty weeks. In the past, it was conventional to classify any baby weighing less than 2500 grams

(5½ pounds) as being premature. Today, it is recognized that the gestational age of a baby—that is, the length of time in the womb—and the birth weight are two separate but very important factors. A baby born at thirty-eight weeks' gestation may be perfectly normal weighing 2300 grams (5 pounds). But a 2500-gram baby born after forty-two weeks of gestation would be considered small for his gestational age.

For a variety of reasons, some babies suffer from growth retardation while they are still in the mother's womb. Doctors call this intrauterine growth retardation, and they use a simple weight/length ratio to help determine whether a small or unusually thin baby is suffering from this condition.

How to Calculate Your Newborn's Weight/Length Ratio

A handheld calculator speeds up these steps. Fill in the blanks with your calculations.

1. Start with your newborn's weight at birth in grams. If you only know your baby's weight in pounds and ounces, convert this figure to ounces (16 ounces to the pound) and multiply the total ounces by 28.5 to get weight in grams. _____

2. Multiply the baby's weight in grams by 100. _____

3. Calculate the baby's length in centimeters. (Do this by multiplying the length in inches by 2.54.) _____

4. Cube the number you arrived at in Step 3. (To cube a number, multiply the number by itself

three times. For example: 3 cubed would be $3 \times 3 \times 3 = 27$.) _____

5. Take the figure you arrived at in Step 2 and divide this by the figure you arrived at in Step 4 (Step 2 ÷ Step 4). The result is your baby's weight/length ratio. For full-term babies, this figure ranges from 2.25 to 3.1. _____

A weight/length ratio of less than 2.25 indicates an unusually thin baby who may be suffering from intrauterine growth retardation. Such a baby would receive special attention in the hospital. At the other extreme is the infant with a weight/length ratio greater than 3.1. Such infants are often born to diabetic mothers but soon begin to follow normal growth patterns.

Birth Defects and Abnormalities

Finally, a word or two about birth defects and other abnormalities. Unfortunately, not all babies are entirely normal. One reliable study showed that major defects were present in 2 percent of newborn babies, and at least one minor abnormality was present in almost 15 percent of live births. The definition of what is a major defect and what is a minor defect—and, indeed, the definition of what is an abnormality at all—is a matter of considerable dispute.

Fortunately, a large percentage of abnormalities can be satisfactorily repaired. In one survey, club foot, in which the foot is twisted out of shape or position, accounted for fully 25 percent of the malformations. Most cases of club feet can be successfully treated by the early application of corrective casts. Congenital dislocation of the hip,

discussed earlier in this chapter, is another common abnormality that is easily repaired.

One deformity that is particularly disheartening for parents because of its cosmetic disfigurement is cleft lip and the cleft palate that is often associated with it. Sometimes called "hare lip" because of its resemblance to a rabbit's split lip, this condition is caused by an embryonic failure of the hard (upper) palate to fuse along the midline. This deformity is common enough that excellent surgical procedures have been devised over the years for almost perfect restoration. A series of operations are performed in several stages at various ages, and most children end up with a totally normal upper lip or, at worst, a slight flattening of the upper lip on one side.

Malformations of the heart also occur with fairly high frequency, and most of these can now be satisfactorily repaired using sophisticated surgical procedures. Many blue babies once destined for certain death can now look forward to long lives.

Malformations of the intestine and related organs can generally be corrected as well. One common problem found most frequently in first-born male infants is pyloric stenosis, which is a partial closure of the outlet of the stomach. Careful examination often reveals an olive-size lump high in the midline of the infant's abdomen. The discovery of such a lump is often preceded by projectile vomiting—that is, vomiting where the material is expelled with great force. Surgical repair of this problem is relatively simple and rapid.

If your baby is born at home, it is important to be certain that blood samples are submitted for screening examinations to detect hidden diseases that are not readily apparent at birth—such as PKU (phenylketonuria), a genetic disease that leaves the body unable to use an essential food element, and inborn absence of the thyroid gland. If left untreated for more than a short time, these disorders lead to severe mental retardation. If treated promptly, however, the child is likely to have normal or very nearly normal intelligence. Many states provide free blood screening examinations for all newborn infants; the doctor or midwife attending your delivery should be able to recommend such a program.

There are some disorders that, unfortunately, cannot be corrected. Among these are the chromosome abnormalities such as Down's syndrome, or mongolism, and deformities involving the spinal cord—most notably, the condition known as spina bifida. This malformation of the spinal cord leaves the nerves that provide feeling and motion to the lower half of the body totally disrupted. Most chromosome disorders and major spinal cord abnormalities can be diagnosed early enough in the pregnancy so that a decision about continuing it or not can be made.

CHAPTER 2

HOW TO EXAMINE YOUR BABY'S SKIN

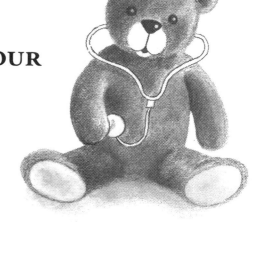

A baby's skin is a standard of perfection. "Baby soft, baby smooth" is the promise of countless powders, creams, and lotions. Everybody wants skin like a baby's.

The fact is, however, that despite the irresistable smoothness and softness of their skin, babies are susceptible to most of the same skin conditions as the rest of us, plus a few of their own. Sooner or later, every baby will have to endure some kind of rash, pimple, bump, or blemish. For this reason, it is important for you to know the nature of baby skin, how to recognize the ailments it may fall heir to, and what you can do when problems arise.

The Structure and Functions of the Skin

The skin is composed of three layers. The top layer, called the epidermis, is the layer you see. The outermost cells of the epidermis are actually dead cells that constantly dry and fall off. These cells are replaced by others from underneath that migrate

to the surface in a process that goes on continuously. New cells are produced at the bottom of the epidermis and slowly die, flatten out, and move to the surface of the skin. The full cycle takes a little less than a month, which means that the outer layer of skin is replaced about twelve times a year. Both the hair and the fingernails, by the way, are also made of dead epidermal cells that have undergone special changes.

The epidermis also contains specialized cells called *melanocytes* that produce the pigments that color the skin. People with dark skin have a large number of melanocytes, whereas those with fair skin have fewer or inactive ones. Ultraviolet rays of the sun induce the melanocytes to step up production of pigment as protection against the sun's rays, which results in tanning. Freckles, too, are produced by melanocytes.

The middle layer of the skin, called the corium or dermis, is the thickest of the three layers. It contains the hair follicles, blood vessels, nerves, muscles, and sweat glands. In babies, this middle layer of skin is not as tightly bound to the upper layer

15

as it will be later on. Thus it's easier for these layers to separate and form a blister. Inflammation can do this. So can rough handling, such as ripping off an adhesive bandage with a heavy hand.

Below the epidermis and the dermis lies the third and final layer of skin. This is a layer of fat that acts as a cushion and shock absorber for the skin and separates it from the underlying muscle and bone. Together, all three layers of your baby's skin are a mere one millimeter thick at birth—about one twenty-fifth of an inch.

The skin acts as a protective envelope for the body and performs a number of vital metabolic functions. The most important of these functions is the maintenance of body temperature. When it is warm or when the body is generating a lot of heat, blood is shunted to the surface of the skin, giving it a pinkish hue. Perspiration is secreted and, as it evaporates, cooling occurs. When it is cold, blood is shunted away from the skin, and the body takes advantage of the insulating value of its underlying layer of fat.

Beyond this, the skin also prevents loss of vital fluids and other substances from within the body, protects against the damaging effects of ultraviolet rays from the sun, helps prevent germs from entering the body, and produces the essential vitamin D. Given its wide array of functions, it is not surprising that trauma that destroys as little as 10 percent of this vital organ has serious medical consequences.

Assessing Your Baby's Skin

Normal baby skin is taken for granted by most parents. It's the rashes and bumps that get all the attention. But even if your baby's skin seems completely unremarkable (other than for its loveliness),

there are still a number of important observations that you should make.

There are five qualities to consider when assessing your baby's skin: color, temperature, texture, moisture, and turgor.

COLOR. Normal color ranges from milky white to deep pink, copper, brown, olive, and bluish tints depending on the baby's genetic background. Become familiar with your baby's normal color. Changes in skin color should be investigated.

TEMPERATURE. Place your hands on different areas of your baby's skin. Compare skin temperature symmetrically—one arm or leg versus the other arm or leg—and from top to bottom. The temperature of your baby's skin should feel about the same over all parts of the body. Know what the skin feels like when baby's body temperature is normal and baby is healthy and comfortable.

TEXTURE. Skin texture of infants and children should be smooth to the touch. You have probably done it many times, but stroke your baby and be aware of this very distinctive feel.

MOISTURE. Your baby's skin should be slightly dry to the touch; it should not feel clammy.

TURGOR. Turgor (rhymes with *burger*) refers to the pliant, elastic quality of normal, healthy skin. Gently grasp the skin of your baby's abdomen between your thumb and forefinger, then release it. Normal skin is elastic and will snap back almost instantly when you let go. When skin turgor has been lost due to dehydration (inadequate fluid intake), the skin remains in a piled-up heap for a few seconds, gradually oozing back to its normal shape instead of springing back promptly. **Poor skin turgor is present only in an ill baby**—one who has been vomiting, has diarrhea, or both. It should be treated as a medical emergency.

Your inspection probably turned up a mark of some sort that does not fit your idea of normal. (Indeed, it would be surprising if you found nothing of note.) Your obvious questions are, of course, what kind of a mark is it and what does it mean?

Your first step toward answering these questions involves describing your finding. That, however, may be trickier than you think. It's next to impossible to talk about skin problems using a lay person's vocabulary. There are many different kinds of bumps, rashes, and other skin phenomena, and you can't describe them all as "red and nasty."

But if you know the difference between a macule and a vesicle, for instance, or a nodule and a bulla, you will be speaking the same language as the doctor. This means you can report your baby's skin problems and subsequent changes to the doctor in more meaningful terms. And you will be better able to understand the doctor's explanations as well.

A Glossary of Terms for Skin Blemishes

BRUISE. A bluish, red, or yellow area that results from small blood vessels having been broken under the skin. The result of a fall or a blow, for example.

BULLA. A fluid-filled, raised area on the skin that is bigger than a quarter of an inch. A blister is an example of a bulla.

CRUST. The dried accumulation of pus, dead skin, and debris that can be found around any wound or abrasion. A scab is an example of a crust.

ERYTHEMA. A reddened area. Sunburn is an example of erythema.

FISSURE. A split in the skin that appears to be quite deep. Chapped lips, for example, produce fissures.

MACULE. A flat area, less than a quarter of an inch across, in which a color change has taken place. The color may be white, brown, purple, or red. Skin texture remains the same. Only the color has changed. Freckles and measle spots are examples of macules.

NODULE. Most people would describe a nodule simply as a lump. It seems to be located deep in the skin, in the middle or underlying layer, rather than on top.

PAPULE. A small raised area that is less than a quarter of an inch across and seems to exist mostly above the skin surface. A wart is an example of a papule.

PATCH. A flat area of color change that is larger than a quarter of an inch in diameter (as opposed to a macule, which is smaller). Flat birthmarks are examples of patches.

PLAQUE. When referring to skin, as opposed to dental plaque, this is a solid, flat-topped, slightly raised area greater than a quarter of an inch in diameter. It may be discolored or the same color as the surrounding skin. Cradle cap, crusts, or psoriasis are examples of plaque.

PUSTULE. If a papule (see Papule) becomes filled with white, puslike fluid, it then becomes a pustule. A pimple is a pustule.

SCALE. Flakes of dry, dead tissue being shed from the skin. Peeling skin and dandruff are examples of scale.

URTICARIA. A flat, slightly raised, itchy red patch that lasts for a half hour or an hour and then disappears. Hives, for example.

VESICLE. If a papule (see Papule) contains clear or yellowish fluid, it is then called a vesicle. A small blister is a vesicle.

WHEAL. An irregularly shaped area, usually flat-topped, that is filled with fluid. It has a much thicker covering than either a vesicle or bulla, and results from a collection of fluid in the deep layers of the skin. Mosquito bites are examples of wheals.

Describing a Skin Condition

The previous glossary is only a sampling of the vocabulary that doctors use to describe skin problems. A parent, of course, would not be expected to command the vocabulary of a dermatologist when reporting a skin problem. But the more precisely you can describe a skin condition, the better. A good close look can yield valuable information as to the type of lesion or mark, the extent of the problem, and whether it is itchy, tender, or numb. And thinking carefully about what your child has been into, eating, or exposed to recently is essential to any diagnosis, including the doctor's.

There are five things to look at when describing a skin condition: the lesion itself, the area involved, the pattern of involvement, the associated symptoms, and the history of the problem.

THE LESION. Any area of skin that differs from normal skin might be called a lesion. Lesions can be anything from patches and scales to bumps, lumps, and bites. As you may have gathered from the glossary, lesions come in all sizes, shapes, and colors. But you can zero in on the salient points by answering the following questions. (A magnifying glass is helpful in these close observations.) Is the lesion flat or raised? Is it circular or irregu-

larly shaped? Is it solid or fluid-filled? If fluid-filled, is the fluid white, clear, or yellow? How would you describe its color? Is the lesion weepy or dry? Is it scaling and flaking?

THE AREA INVOLVED. Determine whether the skin problem is local—confined to one area, such as an arm, leg, or the diaper area, or is general—a rash over most of the body. If localized, note the area involved.

THE PATTERN OF INVOLVEMENT. A telltale pattern can be a strong clue in diagnosing some skin afflictions. Poison ivy, for example, usually shows a streaky pattern—lines of lesions where the irritating oil has been brushed across the skin. Other patterns might be described as clusters of lesions, a widening circle, and so on.

THE ASSOCIATED SYMPTOMS. Look for other symptoms that may accompany a skin problem. The most common of these, of course, is itching. Is the baby scratching or rubbing the lesions? Other symptoms you might find include tenderness, lessened sensation or numbness, redness, fever, and enlarged lymph nodes. And does the baby appear ill?

THE HISTORY OF THE PROBLEM. Time and again, it is the history of the condition that yields the most valuable clues for a diagnosis, and skin problems are no exception. The history of a skin condition includes factors such as a possible allergic reaction to a newly introduced food or medication; an allergic reaction to pollen or pet dander; recent activities that may have brought your child in contact with biting insects, poisonous plants, or toxic chemicals; and, finally, the possibility that your child has been exposed to a playmate's contagious illness. Ask yourself, Where has he been? What might he have gotten into? What has he been eating? What drugs has he been taking? What time of year is it? Has he been playing with children who have since taken sick?

Skin problems and their underlying causes can be difficult to pin down, even for the specialists. Some of them, like diaper rash, are easily diagnosed and dealt with at home. Others, like birthmarks, have little medical consequence. Some, like measles, are easy to identify but require a doctor's attention anyway. Then there are those puzzling rashes that challenge even the specialists. So, except for the simple and obvious problems, skin conditions should be evaluated by a physician.

The following summary will help you to assemble your findings and put them in order. Whenever your baby has a puzzling or worrisome episode of skin trouble, make a list of your findings and take the information with you to the doctor. That way, you won't forget to mention any relevant details.

A Skin Problem Summary

1. Describe the lesion. Check as many conditions as apply.

   ☐ flat   ☐ raised   ☐ circular   ☐ irregular

   ☐ weepy   ☐ dry   ☐ scaling   ☐ crusty

   ☐ fluid-filled   ☐ white fluid

   ☐ yellow fluid   ☐ clear

   Describe the color of the lesion: _____

2. What area of the skin is involved?

   ☐ localized to the following area(s): _____

   ☐ over most of the body

3. Pattern of involvement.

   ☐ a single lesion   ☐ a rash of lesions

   ☐ streaks or lines   ☐ patches

   ☐ other (describe it): _____

   _____

4. Associated symptoms. Check as many symptoms as apply.

   ☐ itchiness   ☐ surrounding redness

   ☐ tenderness   ☐ numbness

   ☐ fever   ☐ enlarged lymph nodes

   Describe how the baby is feeling and acting:

   _____

   _____

   _____

5. History. Check any possibilities.

   ☐ new foods eaten

   ☐ recent new medications

   ☐ contact with animals

   ☐ contact with chemicals

   ☐ use of new salves, powders, or lotions

   ☐ contact with persons with contagious infections or similar symptoms

   Other observations or comments:

   _____

   _____

   _____

Identifying Birthmarks

Fully half of all newborns display some sort of birthmark. There are several varieties of birthmarks, but they all fall into one of two categories: capillary hemangiomas and areas of heavy pigmentation.

Capillary Hemangiomas

STORK BITE. Capillary hemangiomas are collections of small blood vessels—capillaries—just under the surface of the skin. The so-called stork bite falls into this category. These flat pink marks occur most frequently over the eyelids, the bridge of the nose, and the back of the neck. Those over the eyelid usually clear by one year, whereas those over the bridge of the nose persist a bit longer. The ones on the back of the neck usually clear up also, although there are some that persist as a minor discoloration into adult life.

PORT-WINE STAIN. A port-wine stain is a darker and more extensive kind of capillary hemangioma, compared to the small pink stork bite. Port-wine stains usually occur on one side of the face or on an extremity and, unfortunately, are most permanent in nature, though they do fade somewhat.

STRAWBERRY MARK. A third sort of red birthmark is a raised, red, rubbery nodule with a roughened surface called a strawberry mark. Sometimes these are not present at birth but develop at two to four weeks of age. These strawberry marks persist somewhat longer than stork bites but do eventually fade. Half of all strawberry marks are gone by age five, about three-fourths by age seven, and about 90 percent by age

nine. Virtually all strawberry marks clear up by the time of adolescence.

Since all of these capillary hemangiomas are caused by collections of tiny blood vessels just under the skin, you can easily check to see if a red mark on your baby is a birthmark or a bruise.

How to Identify Capillary Hemangiomas

1. Press down on the mark with the bottom of an ordinary water glass—one you can see through.

2. Hold the glass pressed on the mark for a few seconds and observe the mark through the glass. If there is some blanching, or whitening, of the red mark where you press down, you are looking at an area of skin filled with tiny blood vessels—a hemangioma, in other words. This blanching is more difficult to see in dark-skinned babies because the pigment in the skin partially obscures the hemangioma.

3. If the color does not blanch when you press down, it is probably a small bruise.

Areas of Heavy Pigmentation

Areas of heavy pigmentation are caused by a clustering of the pigment cells that give skin its color—the melanocytes. Where these melanocytes happen to cluster together, it shows as a dark spot on the surface of the skin.

MONGOLIAN SPOTS. Mongolian spots appear on about 90 percent of all dark-skinned babies. These bluish-gray, flat birthmarks occur most commonly over the back and buttocks, although they can be found on any part of the body. They vary greatly in size and shape. Mongolian spots usually disappear in the first few years of life, though they occasionally persist into adulthood.

CAFÉ AU LAIT SPOTS. Brown areas of pigment, often called café au lait spots, are found in about 10 percent of light-skinned babies and roughly 25 percent of dark-skinned infants. They are light brown on light skin (coffee with milk, as the name suggests) and darker brown on dark skin. They are generally oval and range in size from less than a quarter of an inch in diameter to an inch or more. Unlike mongolian spots, café au lait spots persist throughout life. They are harmless, but the presence of six or more café au lait spots greater than five-eighths of an inch in diameter may be associated with a more serious condition called neurofibromatosis. These are many small fibrous growths along certain nerve tracts. If you find your baby has six or more café au lait spots, bring this to the attention of your doctor.

MOLES. Pigment cells in clusters are also responsible for moles. Moles are brown, tan, or black spots, usually more or less circular, which first begin to appear on the skin at about one year of age. They may be flat or slightly raised. As time goes by, children generally develop more moles; most adults have twenty or more. Moles are generally harmless, but if any of the following events occur they should be called to the attention of your doctor:

- If a mole increases in size
- If the mole bleeds, crusts, or develops an ulcer or sore
- If the mole becomes irregular in shape

- If a mole becomes rough in texture
- If a mole changes color. Particularly dangerous is the addition of red, white, or blue coloration to a brown or black mole.

Moles in the genital area or at clothing pressure points where they receive continual chafing should be evaluated by a physician. Do not remove moles at home by any method. It must be done by a physician.

FRECKLES. Freckles are yet another form in which skin pigment manifests itself. These are small pigmented spots, caused by overly active pigment cells. They are generally brought out by sunlight in summer and fade somewhat in winter. They are most commonly seen on the face but also appear on the neck and shoulders. Fair-skinned people have the most freckles, and a heavily freckled parent can pass along the tendency to a child.

Freckles cannot be prevented, even by sunscreen lotion. Lemon juice does not bleach them. If freckles appear, the best thing you can do is help your child learn to live with them by referring to them, if at all, as being particularly attractive.

Identifying Rashes and Inflammations

Dermatitis is a very general word used to refer to many kinds of skin ailments. It means, simply, an inflammation of the skin. There are many causes of dermatitis, the most common of which are allergic reactions and contact with irritating substances. Frequently, however, the cause of dermatitis cannot be pinned down. The following are some of the most common.

Milia

Milia shows up on nearly half of all newborn babies. Milia consists of tiny white bumps over the baby's nose and cheeks, and less commonly on the forehead and chin. Although these little pimples contain white material, the material is not pus and the pimples are not infected. The pimples result from blocked skin pores, and the white material is an accumulation of normally secreted material. These pores will open spontaneously at one to two months of age. Harsh scrubbing is not recommended, nor should creams or skin lotions be used in an attempt to clear the condition more rapidly than its normal one- to two-month course.

Erythema Toxicum

About half of all babies develop a red, blotchy rash on the second or third day of life. The blotches are about half an inch in diameter, with a small white lump in the center (a papule or vesicle). This is called erythema toxicum. The rash can occur on any area of the body, and in a few babies the lesions can be quite numerous. The cause of this dermatitis is unknown, but it always clears up without treatment by the age of one week or sooner.

Face Rash

Within the first few months of life, most babies develop a face rash. This may be due to an irritation from drooling or from a food-acid mixture that has been regurgitated from the stomach. Some rashes develop for no reason that is immediately apparent. Wipe the baby's face frequently. Protect the face with a light application of a non-oily skin cream, such as hand lotion, and allow the baby to

sleep with its head on a cloth diaper or other moisture-absorbing surface.

Heat Rash

In warm, humid weather, many babies develop heat rash, which is characterized by pinpoint pink bumps (papules) most commonly seen on the neck and chest and is caused by blocked sweat glands.

Heat rash will clear up in two to three days if the skin is kept cool. This can be accomplished with cool baths given every two to three hours, or with air conditioning, or with the breeze of an electric fan. Dress your baby as lightly as possible. Calamine lotion may be useful, but avoid ointments since they can keep the sweat glands blocked and simply make matters worse. Sterile baby corn starch may be helpful.

Cradle Cap

Cradle cap (seborrheic dermatitis) is another common inflammation of the skin that affects about 50 percent of infants shortly after birth. Its cause is unknown. Cradle cap consists of yellow, oily scales and crusts on the scalp.

Mild cases are best treated by shampooing daily and by carefully brushing the yellow, oily scales and crusts from the scalp. Be gentle but persistent; you will not injure the baby's fontanels. If the scalp is very crusty, soften the crusty parts by applying baby oil an hour before shampooing. Ask your pharmacist to recommend a shampoo that works well for cradle cap; there are several on the market. When the head is fully lathered, use a soft brush on the scales and be persistent. Once the condition is cleared, it is no longer necessary to use a special shampoo or to pre-treat the baby's scalp with baby oil. Regular shampooing with baby shampoo two or three times a week should be adequate to prevent recurrences. But if the condition becomes red, weepy, or raw, or if it involves the eyelids or the ear canal consult the doctor.

Diaper Rash

Skin inflammations caused by contact with an irritating substance are known as contact dermatitis. Diaper rash is by far the most common kind of contact dermatitis in babies. In this case, the irritating substance can be urine and feces, detergents and fabric softeners, ointments and other substances applied to the diaper area (including the disposable wet towels some parents use to clean the diaper area), or any combination of these. Occasionally a fungus infection will complicate things.

A diaper rash is simply a large, reddened, sometimes cracked area of skin in the diaper area, particularly around the groin and between the legs. Usually the rash is mild, but sometimes it can become quite severe. A severe rash is a darker beet red in color and quite extensive. Sometimes pimples, boils, and yellow crusting is present. In circumcised boys, there may occasionally be a scab on the tip of the penis. If any of these conditions occur, or if the child has a thrush infection in the mouth (see Chapter 8, "How to Examine Your Baby's Mouth and Teeth"), the baby should be taken to see the doctor the next day.

In the absence of blistering or any other complications, most diaper rashes can be treated very satisfactorily at home. The key to treating diaper rash is drying. The longer you can keep your baby out of diapers each day, the faster the rash will clear. A baby with diaper rash should sleep without diapers, on absorbent padding. A towel or cloth diaper is useful for this. When you do diaper your baby, use single-layer cloth diapers and do not double diaper. Air circulation is important. Also, do not use plastic-covered disposable diapers; they keep moisture against the skin and prevent adequate drying. You should not put plastic pants over cloth diapers for the same reason. Change the baby frequently. While cloth diapers are inconvenient, you will find them useful while combating diaper rash.

Avoid using a heat lamp to dry up the rash. The risk of prolonged exposure makes this far too dangerous. An ordinary desk lamp with a 60-watt bulb at a distance of about two feet can provide a small amount of heat without harm, but it is usually unnecessary if the baby can go without diapers for fairly long periods of time during the day.

Wash diaper rash with plain water; mild soap is needed only for cleanups after bowel movements. When you do use soap, be sure to rinse the area thoroughly. Apply a thin film of a lotion three times a day after washings to keep the skin well hydrated, but keep the surface dry. A thin coating of zinc oxide ointment, which is available without prescription, may be even more effective. Ask your doctor or pharmacist for a recommendation of a lotion to use.

With proper treatment, considerable improvement should be noticed within three days. If you are keeping the baby's skin dry and using the other measures suggested above, but the diaper rash does not show rapid improvement in three or four days, then you should consult your doctor right away.

Poison Ivy

Another kind of contact dermatitis children often get is poison ivy. Typically, a child is playing outside in a field or woods. Within a day or two, a rash begins to develop on exposed parts of the body—the hands, arms, feet, and legs. Sometimes the face, groin, and abdomen are affected, but rarely the back. The rash is due to skin sensitivity to the minute amount of oil transferred to the skin from contact with the poison ivy plant. Once the child has touched the plant, he may transfer the sensitizing oil from his hands to his face or other parts of the body. The irritating oil can also be transferred to a child's skin from the fur of a dog or cat that has come in contact with the plant.

The first signs of poison ivy are redness and some initial blistering. In two to three days, the blisters break, exuding a yellowish fluid that dries on the surface of the body, leaving yellow crusting. Poison ivy lesions appear in streaks for two reasons: usually the child brushes against the plant and the sensitizing fluid is deposited in streaks; then the child may have some of the fluid on his nails or fingers and transfer streaks of it to almost any part of the body. The outbreak does not erupt all at once. Several days may elapse between the first evidence of a rash and the appearance of the final blisters.

Poison ivy can usually be managed at home with cold water soaks, calamine lotion, Benadryl and other itch-relief creams, and the new cortisone creams available without prescription. The sooner you begin treatment, the better. In younger children, cut the fingernails quite short to minimize scratching. The rash takes a good ten to fourteen days to run its course. If your child has an extensive case of poison ivy, particularly if it involves the face or eyes, take him to the doctor immediately.

The best treatment for poison ivy, of course, is prevention. Once you know your child is sensitive to poison ivy, teach him to identify the characteristic three-leafed plant, even if you have to learn about it yourself first from a book about plants or from a knowledgeable person. Poison ivy and its close relative poison oak both have the characteristic three-leaf clusters. The plant can grow as either a low or tallish shrub, as a trailing vine, or as a climber, so don't rule out any of these forms. The three-leaf configuration is the key. All parts of the plant are poisonous in all seasons. Smoke from burning the plant is also toxic.

If you believe your child has been exposed to poison ivy, wash him immediately with a strong laundry soap such as Fels Naptha. Mild bath soaps are far less effective for this purpose. If done within one-half to one hour after exposure, you may be able to remove the sensitizing oils and prevent the rash. Be sure not to get alkaline soaps in the child's eyes.

Poison ivy oils may cling to clothing for weeks. Therefore, all clothing the child was wearing at the time of exposure should be thoroughly washed to prevent further infection.

Dandruff

Dandruff is quite normal and does not represent a disease state. It is an exaggeration of a normal process—the continuous shedding and regeneration of skin. On most of the body, flakes of skin simply fall to the ground unnoticed. But on the head, they are apt to become trapped among the hair shafts and accumulate, particularly if the hair tends to be oily. Dandruff is not an infection, and it is not contagious. Your child cannot catch dandruff from anyone.

The main treatment for dandruff is removing the flakes. This is best done by washing the hair daily and brushing it vigorously. Brushing before shampooing will loosen the flakes so that more of them will be washed away, keeping the hair free of dandruff for a somewhat longer period of time.

If dandruff persists or if the scaling is patchy and broken hairs can be seen within the patchy area consult your physician.

Allergic Reactions

Animal products such as wool, feathers, and fur can be allergy-causing irritants. These irritants include common items such as feather pillows and wool sweaters. Chemicals of all kinds can provoke a skin reaction in allergic individuals. The culprits might be synthetic fabrics, the dyes used to color them, metal jewelry (even gold for some people), perfumes, cosmetics, and soaps of all kinds. Certain foods and prescription and nonprescription drugs can produce adverse reactions that are exhibited on the skin. Bee and wasp stings can produce allergic skin eruptions besides the original lump from the bite. An allergic skin reaction can take different forms, including hives and eczema.

HIVES. Hives resemble giant mosquito bites. The classic hive—consisting of a reddened area with a white, sometimes raised center—is called a wheal. Hives usually occur in large numbers and are quite itchy.

Any child who develops hives should be watched closely for difficulty in breathing or swallowing and should be rushed to the doctor or hospital emergency room if either of these symptoms develop.

Children with hives sometimes develop abdominal pains, and these should also be brought to a physician's attention. In fact, most children with moderate to severe hives should be taken to the doctor. If the onset of hives follows the taking of a prescribed drug, tell the doctor at once since it may signal a more serious reaction to come.

The primary treatment of hives consists of antihistamines (the swelling of hives is caused by a histamine, a protein released in response to sensitivity or allergy to some substance). Children with recurrent hives due to known allergies or with extremely mild hives can be treated at home with antihistamines obtained by prescription or from the drugstore on recommendation of a doctor. But be alert for the danger signs noted above.

ECZEMA. Eczema is a term used to describe a series of events that occur on the skin in response to an allergic reaction: redness, swelling, the appearance of small, fluid-filled vesicles (tiny blisters), weeping, oozing, scaling, and crusting.

Eczema tends to be a chronic condition—clearing and later flaring up again for many years. Some thickening of the skin and deepening of normal skin markings may occur over time in response to chronic rubbing and scratching. Early treatment of itching may help forestall a more severe attack. A child with eczema in an active state should be bathed once a day, but no soap should be used in the area of the rash—soap is likely to aggravate the condition. Children with eczema usually have dry skin, and a moisturizer will help keep their skin well hydrated.

Once a moderate to severe rash actually develops, cortisone-type creams are the mainstay of treatment. Any child with eczema, however, should be under a doctor's care. The doctor will suggest various ways to relieve itching and prevent infections, and will try to discover what food or other substance is causing the allergy.

Identifying Skin Infections

The skin is alive with microorganisms—bacteria, viruses, and fungi. Practically all are harmless, and some even help control populations of potentially harmful bacteria. Some, however, will invade the skin and cause a variety of infections. Most healthy babies and children can fight them off, but no one is immune to them. Children suffering from other kinds of illness are especially vulnerable to these common skin infections.

Impetigo

Impetigo is a bacterial infection that is very common among toddlers and preschoolers. It begins as a small, flat, reddish area (macule) that soon becomes vesicular (raised and fluid-filled). The vesicles rupture and the yellowish fluid that is released dries to form heavy, honey-colored crusts. Impetigo is both unsightly and itchy. It is also contagious. If the child scratches the infected area, he may transfer bacteria trapped under his fingernails to another part of the body. He can also infect other children in this way. Direct contact is necessary, however, and children who are simply in the same room as the child with impetigo need not be concerned about becoming infected.

It is best to let a doctor treat impetigo. Oral antibiotics may be necessary, and there are some potentially serious complications. With proper treatment, impetigo should clear up within one to two weeks.

Pimples and Boils

Pimples and boils are also caused by bacteria. Boils sometimes start as small pimples and swell to an angry red bump. They may also start as flat red areas. They are tender, contagious, apt to recur, and may leave scars. For all of these reasons, boils should be seen by a doctor. When a boil is fully developed, he may want to lance it. It takes several days for a boil to develop to a state where it is ready for lancing. During this time, soak the boil with hot

washcloths for a period of twenty minutes four times a day. Sometimes a small boil will resolve satisfactorily with this treatment. If not, the boil will come to a head, and the center will become soft. At this point, it is ready for lancing by the doctor.

Keep the area of the skin around the boil clean while it is being treated with hot soaks. Rubbing alcohol or a mild solution of bleach (a teaspoon of bleach added to a quart of water) are both satisfactory for this purpose.

If your child develops a fever or chills, or if one or more red streaks going away from the boil develop, take him to the doctor immediately.

The treatment of pimples is generally the same as for boils: hot soaks four times a day and cleansing of the area with rubbing alcohol or a mild bleach solution. A pimple may come to a head and rupture by itself under the hot soaks. If this happens, cleanse the area well and apply an antibiotic ointment.

If the pimples seem to be spreading or are numerous, see the doctor. **Do not, under any circumstances, open or squeeze a pimple anywhere around the nose, face, head, or neck.** Squeezing pimples in these areas can cause a very serious brain infection. Do not cover pimples with adhesive bandages or petroleum jelly as this can only make them worse.

Warts

Warts and cold sores are both caused by viruses. Viruses invade body cells and stimulate the host cell to form more virus material.

Warts are easily recognized as dry, round, raised lesions that are brown or gray. If you examine one closely with a magnifying glass, you will notice several very fine indentations on its surface. Warts are common in children and can occur anywhere, but you are most likely to find them on exposed areas such as the hands, face, and soles of the feet.

Like many viral infections, warts follow an unpredictable course. If left untreated, most warts usually disappear in about two years. Various treatments may speed up this process. For reasons that are not understood, warts seem to be psychosuggestible. That means, if you think some treatment is going to make your warts go away, chances are it will work.

Preparations containing salicylic acid are usually effective. Ask your pharmacist for suggestions. Paint the substance on the surface of the wart once daily. The surface of the wart gradually turns into dead skin. File this off with an emery board so that the next application of salicylic acid can work on living tissue. However, don't file so much or so vigorously as to make it bleed.

Warts are mildly contagious and picking at warts may cause them to spread. If your child makes one of his warts bleed, the blood, if left dried on the skin, may cause another wart to develop. Warts that seem to be multiplying or that persist for more than a few months, or warts on the bottom of the feet (plantar warts) should be seen by a doctor.

Cold Sores

Cold sores, also called fever blisters, are painful blisters that occur on the outer lip. A cold sore is usually small and sometimes crosses the border between the lip and the facial skin. Because it is painful, it may interfere with a child's eating. Cold sores are caused by the herpes simplex virus, type I. This is *not* the virus that causes genital herpes.

If your child develops a cold sore for the first time, take him to see the doctor promptly. There are medications with specific activity against the herpes virus that may cut down the length of time the cold sore is present. But even without this ointment, cold sores heal completely within one to two weeks. Application of alcohol four times daily will help speed the healing process somewhat.

The herpes virus tends to come and go mysteriously, lying dormant inside a cell for long periods of time and then causing another outbreak. Children who are prone to develop them may find that recurrences seem to be triggered by exposure to sunlight. A sunscreen lotion may help a bit in these cases.

Ringworm

Along with bacteria and viruses, certain funguses (fungi) can also invade the skin. There are many fungus infections, but the one children get most often is ringworm. Ringworm (not a worm at all) looks like an irregular, round pink patch with a raised scaly ring around the edge of the pink area. Once established, it usually increases in size. The center of the ring clears as the scaly red edge creeps outward.

Small areas of ringworm on the body (not the scalp)—fewer than three spots—usually can be handled at home. It is treated with antifungal agents. Several of these are available without prescription and are effective in treating small ringworm lesions that do not involve the scalp or hair. Apply the cream four times daily and try to keep your child from rubbing or scratching the patches. Continue the treatment for one week after the lesion seems to be gone. Ringworm is only very slightly contagious, and there is no reason to keep your child away from other children if he develops this problem. After forty-eight hours of treatment, it is not the least bit contagious.

Ringworm of the scalp and hair *cannot* be treated at home. If the scalp or hair is involved, if there are more than three patches on the body, or if treatment of minor cases with a nonprescription cream does not help within two weeks, consult the doctor.

Hair and Nail Problems

Children's hair varies with genetic factors, so it may be straight or curly, coarse or fine. But the distinguishing feature of normal hair in children is that it is silky, strong, elastic, and shiny. Normal fingernails and toenails are pink, rounded, smooth, hard, and flexible. The color, of course, will be darker or lighter depending on your child's complexion.

Any changes from a normal condition that cannot be easily explained should be called to the attention of a physician. Easily explained changes would be nails that are broken while playing or hair that is bleached by the sun. You should check with your doctor when hair loses color for no reason, falls out, or becomes stringy, dry, and brittle. Nails that are chipped, broken, furrowed, flaky, or otherwise unusual looking should be seen by a doctor. There may be a very simple explanation for these events—a minor fungal infection, for example—but it may also indicate a more serious systemic problem involving the parathyroid or adrenal glands. A doctor should be the one to decide what the condition is.

Childhood Diseases That Show on the Skin

There are four common childhood diseases that are systemic (affecting the whole body) and are characterized by a very obvious rash: roseola, chicken pox, measles, and scarlet fever. All of them are highly contagious.

Roseola

Roseola occurs in children between the ages of six months and three years. It is characterized by a fine, pinkish red rash, predominantly on the trunk, and it is much less obvious or is absent on the legs, arms, and face.

Typically, the child develops a high fever for two to four days. Usually the doctor is unable to find any specific reason for the fever. The fever then disappears quickly, and within twenty-four hours the rash appears. During the time when the high fever is present, the child appears to be only mildly ill. The rash that follows lasts only a day or two. Other children who have been in contact with your child during the febrile period or while he has the rash may contract it too. Once the rash is gone, the disease is no longer contagious. The incubation period—that is, from the time of exposure to the appearance of the first symptoms—is about twelve days.

No treatment is necessary for roseola. You need only call your doctor if the rash becomes deep purple, if deep purple splotches develop in it, or if the rash lasts more than three days. If the child is unusually ill, of course, you should contact the doctor. If the fever that precedes the rash is very high, your doctor should be informed and the child watched for signs of progressing illness. Cooling baths may be prescribed along with age-appropriate doses of acetaminophen or ibuprofen.

Chicken Pox

The rash associated with chicken pox consists of small red bumps that develop into little watery blisters. These break to become open sores and, finally, dry crusted lesions. The sores appear in crops, and the diagnosis of chicken pox is made by finding lesions in all states of development, from the early red bump to the dry crusted pox. New eruptions continue to appear on a daily basis for four or five days.

Chicken pox is a contagious disease, and your child must be kept out of school and away from other children. Do not take a child with chicken pox to the doctor's office as you will simply expose everyone else in the office to the disease. It remains contagious until about seven days after the onset of the disease, or until all the old lesions have crusted over and no new ones are appearing. Chicken pox is not contagious for those who have already had the disease.

The main treatment for chicken pox is to relieve the itching. Trim your child's fingernails as short as possible to discourage scratching and infection of the crusted pox lesions. A cool bath every three or four hours is helpful. Bathing does not cause the rash to spread. Calamine lotion may help relieve the itching as does Benadryl itch-relief cream. Acetaminophen (Tylenol, for example) may also make your child more comfortable. **Do not give aspirin.**

Chicken pox sores may also occur in the mouth, in which case the child may not be the least bit interested in food. Be sure he gets enough to drink during this time. Any liquid will do, but apple juice or milk will be more soothing than citric juices.

Infected chicken pox lesions may turn into impetigo, the bacterial infection discussed earlier in this chapter. Call your doctor if the sores look as though they are becoming infected, if your child cannot sleep because of the itching, or if your child develops a fever, becomes confused, or develops a headache or a stiff neck.

Immunization against chicken pox is now available and a recommended addition to the list of childhood inoculations.

Measles

Most children these days are immunized against both measles and German measles (rubella); thus, rashes caused by these two diseases are not often seen. Measles and German measles cause a flat, blotchy-red rash that starts on the face and spreads downward over the entire body. Other symptoms include red eyes, a runny nose, and a cough. If you suspect your child has measles, you should take him to your doctor promptly. Complications from measles can be dangerous and even life-threatening.

Scarlet Fever

Scarlet fever is another systemic disease that causes a rash. It is caused by streptococcus bacteria—the same organisms that cause strep throat—and is characterized by a reddened, sunburn-like rash that is most prominent over the chest and abdomen, and less so on the arms and legs. The redness may be more pronounced in the skin folds, particularly in the groin and at the bend in the arm. The skin sometimes has a slightly rough texture, the face may be flushed, and the area around the mouth may appear unusually pale. Other symptoms include a sore throat and a significant fever. Your child will probably act as though she is not feeling well.

All children with scarlet fever should be seen by a doctor. Do not attempt home treatment. **Untreated, scarlet fever may lead to both heart and kidney disease.**

Skin Problems Caused by Insects

Babies and small children are particularly vulnerable to insect infestations, bites, and stings. Their health habits are not as fastidious as an adult's, nor are their swatting skills as well developed. Parents can help by insisting that children wear shoes, by not dressing them in bright clothing, and by not using perfumed shampoos and other scented grooming products during insect-heavy months. Use insect repellents without deet (N,N-diethyl-meta-toluamide; read the label) and be sure to keep them away from the child's mouth and eyes. Apply any repellent you use sparingly with your hand rather than by creating clouds of spray. During trips to the woods or fields, it's best for the child to wear long sleeves and long trousers.

Recognizing Insect Bites and Stings

Bloodsucking insects, such as mosquitoes and gnats, inject a foreign protein that makes it easier for them to suck blood. This causes itching, which, in turn, prompts the victim to scratch. The result is a firm papule that may be capped by a fluid-filled vesicle. Red scratch lines may be present. Treatment consists of anti-itch medications. Keep the area clean to avoid secondary infections.

Bees, wasps, hornets, and other stinging insects inject a venom that causes a small red area with a wheal and itching. Remove the stinger if it is still there and you can get at it easily; clean the area with soap and water, and apply ice. If your child is hypersensitive to insect stings, the whole body may react to the venom with symptoms such as generalized pain and skin eruptions over the whole body, even in the mouth. There could also be nausea, vomiting, confusion, and difficulty breathing. **Any such allergic reaction is an emergency that requires immediate medical attention.**

Scabies

Some insects don't just eat and run; they are parasites that take up residence on the body. Two of the most common of these are scabies and lice.

Scabies and lice occur most often in crowded, unsanitary conditions. They can be passed among people in close-contact situations.

Scabies is an infestation by a small insect called a mite. The infestation is suggested by reddened, raised, irregular lines, particularly about the wrists, ankles, fingerwebs, underarm area, between the legs near the genitals, or, in infants, on the face. These irregular lines are actually the burrows of the female insect as she works her way through the skin.

Scabies requires treatment with an antiparasitic prescription lotion. If your doctor prescribes this for your child, follow directions carefully. Recent studies have shown that some of these ointments can be absorbed into the body and become concentrated in the central nervous system. It should not be applied too often or left on for too long. Usually a single application provides adequate treatment. All clothing and bedding in the household (not just the child's) should be well cleansed and disinfected. Follow doctor's instructions carefully in this regard. The doctor will also suggest a cream or lotion to relieve the itching.

Lice

Infestation with lice is suggested by severe itching at night together with scraped and scratched pimples and pustules. You are most apt to find the lice and their eggs, or nits, in the seams of clothing.

Head lice cause similar sores and itching and are diagnosed by finding tiny white eggs firmly attached to hair shafts near the scalp. Lice infestations are a large problem among school-age children.

Both types of lice are effectively treated with antiparasitic medications: ointments for body lice and shampoos for head lice. If you find either type of lice on your child, contact your doctor promptly since the most effective medications require a prescription and professional instructions for their use. As with scabies, all clothing and bedding (not just the child's) should be thoroughly cleaned.

Sunburn

Sunburn is a generalized redness over exposed areas of the body after substantial time spent in the sun. Because of the natural makeup of the skin, some children burn far more easily than others. In general, blond children burn more easily than brunettes, though some brunettes have very fair skin and burn quite easily, too.

In children over two, you can cut down the inflammatory reaction a bit with a child dosage of ibuprofen, though it won't "cure" a burn. Immediately after exposure, give the child a dose of ibuprofen appropriate for his age (follow label instructions carefully). Four to six hours later, repeat it. Ater repeating it a third time, you will have accomplished all you can this way, and you need not continue giving it.

More conventional sunburn treatments include cold baths and cold soaks. Showers may be painful because of the spray, and soap may be irritating. Do not apply ointments, petroleum jelly, or butter to a sunburn; these greasy substances will simply make the symptoms worse. Nor should you apply first aid anesthetic cream or spray. These often contain benzocaine, and the inflamed skin may become sensitized to this substance; this again will make matters worse.

Very severe sunburn must be treated by a physician. Severe sunburn consists not only of redness but also of extensive blistering. One or two blisters are not particularly significant, but ten or twelve blisters certainly are and should be brought to medical attention. If your child is unable to keep his eyes open or look at lights, this may indicate possible sun damage to the eyes. Heat exhaustion can also be associated with sunburn. A body temperature over 102°F (39°C) and/or fainting suggest this possibility. Any of these findings associated with sunburn should be seen by a doctor.

The best treatment for sunburn is prevention, of course. The most practical means is through the use of a sunscreen lotion. Most sunscreen products display a sun protection factor (SPF) number from two up; the higher the number, the greater the degree of protection. Use a relatively high SPF number on fair-skinned children The child should develop some tan, however, to prevent further burning should he go outside without sunscreen protection. It is better to use a substance that will let some, but not all, of the sun's rays through.

CHAPTER 3

HOW TO CHECK YOUR BABY'S HEART, LUNGS, AND VITAL SIGNS

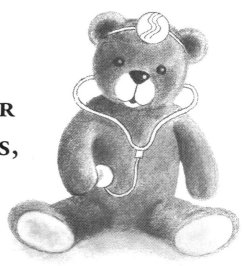

Your baby's heart is, in essence, a simple pump with a straightforward function—that of circulating blood throughout the body. Blood carries nutrients and oxygen to body cells and picks up waste products for disposal. The body's source of oxygen is the air, of course, which the lungs take in like a set of bellows. Together, the heart and lungs are responsible for three of the four vital signs (discussed later in this chapter) that reveal so much about the body's state of health. So it is important to observe and check these functions.

How the Heart Works

Your baby's heart is a hollow, muscular organ. It is divided in half by a wall, or septum, that runs through the middle of the heart—inside—from top to bottom. Each side has two chambers: a right atrium (entrance chamber) and a right ventricle; a left atrium and a left ventricle. The two sides of the heart work in unison. The right side pumps blood through the lungs, where it gives up carbon dioxide and collects oxygen. The oxygen-rich blood then returns to the left side of the heart, and from there it is pumped to the rest of the body through the arteries. The blood completes its cycle by returning through the veins to the right side of the heart.

Valves shunt the blood through the chambers of the heart in the correct sequence, and a built-in pacemaker keeps the pumping action going at a regular rate. This rhythmic pumping action makes a characteristic "lub-dub" sound that can be heard easily through a stethoscope.

Listening to Your Baby's Heart Using a Stethoscope

Stethoscopes suitable for home use are available in most drugstores. If you purchase a home blood-pressure monitoring kit (a good investment for both parents and children), a stethoscope is usually included in the kit. All stethoscopes consist of two hooked metal tubes fitted with earplugs that rest comfortably inside your ears. These metal tubes are attached to rubber or plastic tubing that is joined by a connector and then continues into a

33

single tube. This section ends in either a flat disc or a bell-shaped piece that is placed against the chest to pick up sounds.

The flat disc generally gives a somewhat louder volume than the bell-shaped piece. In fact, the less expensive stethoscopes intended for home use usually are fitted with only the disc, which is all you need to hear normal heart sounds or to detect basic abnormal sounds. The bell-shaped chest piece is useful for detecting the very lowest tones and for diagnosing variations of heart murmurs, but these are not things you can do yourself anyway.

Note that the ear plugs have a slant to them. Hold the stethoscope in front of you so that the curve or slant of the ear plugs points slightly forward. Now place one of the ear plugs in each ear. Most ear pieces can be rotated a bit until you get the position where they fit snugly and comfortably in your ears.

The area where the heartbeat is most loudly heard is called the point of maximum impulse. This point is located on the left side of the baby's chest, just below the nipple and very slightly toward the center. Place the chest piece of the stethoscope here.

You should now be able to hear the rhythmic beating of your baby's heart. This beating consists of two closely coupled sounds, commonly described as "lub-dub, lub-dub, lub-dub." There should be a short pause between the pairs of sounds where you hear little if anything.

Listen for several moments. Heart sounds should be clear and distinct in quality, with a regular and even rhythm.

Variations in Heart Sounds

It's not uncommon in children for the heart rate to increase upon breathing in and decrease while breathing out. The name for this is sinus arrhythmia, and it's a normal condition that children outgrow. If your child's heartbeat does not sound even and rhythmic, have him hold his breath, if he's old enough to do this. If the heart rate remains steady, then the phenomenon is nothing that should cause you concern.

Abnormal heart sounds are called murmurs. Normally blood flows smoothly through the heart. A murmur is caused by a slightly turbulent blood flow. This turbulence causes a blowing sound that varies in loudness from barely audible to so loud it almost drowns out the normal heart sounds.

The most common murmur, called a systolic murmur, is heard *between* the two major heart sounds—that is, between the lub and the dub. When listening to a child with such a murmur, the heart might sound like this: "lub-shsss-dub, lub-shsss-dub, lub-shsss-dub."

Murmurs that occur *after* the second heart sound are called diastolic murmurs and might sound like this: "lub-dub-shsss, lub-dub-shsss, lub-dub-shsss."

Detecting a murmur is not necessarily a reason for panic. Sometimes, as the heart grows, the blood will flow in a turbulent pattern for several months or even several years. Murmurs caused by these irregularities in heart shape during growth are called physiologic murmurs and generally have little permanent significance. In years gone by, many children were unnecessarily restricted in their activities because "the doctor said they had a heart murmur." Today, a murmur is evaluated carefully by the doctor, and if the verdict is that it's nothing to worry about, then don't worry about it. However, any murmur you detect should be reported to the doctor for evaluation. Don't make your own diagnosis.

Heart Defects

Well before your baby is born, the information a doctor elicits from your health history can provide valuable clues to your baby's potential risk of heart disease. Two factors, inherited traits and conditions during pregnancy, may influence this risk.

During pregnancy, things such as exposure to rubella (German measles) during the first three months of pregnancy, diabetes, and poor nutrition increase the risk that the baby will have a heart problem. Statistics show that babies of older mothers (over forty) seem to be at greater risk. The most important inherited factor is a history of congenital heart defects in the family (that is, defects present at birth). The existence of one or more of these risk factors in no way guarantees that your baby will have a heart problem. It just means that the doctor should pay special attention to this aspect of your infant's health.

Within minutes of your baby's birth, heart function is assessed through two of the five items on the Apgar Test (see Chapter 1). One thing the doctor checks is the number of heartbeats per minute, and another thing is body color—an indication of whether the blood is receiving enough oxygen as it is pumped through the lungs. Serious congenital heart abnormalities are often detected at this point.

Occasionally, a heart defect is not detected at birth. Its symptoms may be so subtle that they become apparent only as the infant grows. At some point, however, the baby's growth and energy expenditures outstrip the heart's capacity to provide oxygenated blood. This happens gradually. But as it does, a baby's activity level will drop off. In order to compensate for the inadequate oxygen supply, she will do less—sit instead of crawl and take frequent rests during play periods. She will eat slowly, often pausing to rest; consequently she will consume less food and not gain the weight she should.

Heart defects provoke great anxiety in parents, sometimes more than is called for, and this anxiety is invariably communicated to the child. Many heart problems can be successfully corrected. So if you think your baby shows signs of heart disease, seek out expert advice. Then follow the doctor's advice carefully without putting restrictions of your own on the child that the doctor doesn't deem necessary.

How the Lungs Work

Your baby's heart shares space in the chest cavity with the lungs. The tip, or apex, of each lung rises just above the collarbone. The broader base of each lung rests on the diaphragm, the partition separating the abdominal cavity from the chest cavity. The diaphragm is a muscular arch located above the stomach, just about where the rib cage starts curving down from the breastbone.

Veins carry blood from the body that is laden with carbon dioxide to the right side of the heart. The blood is then pumped to the lungs, where the carbon dioxide is disposed of. The blood picks up fresh oxygen from air breathed in by the lungs, returns to the left side of the heart, and is then pumped through the arteries to all the cells of the body.

Checking Your Baby's Breathing

Take a few moments when your baby is quiet and simply observe his breathing. This is easiest to do when he is lying on his back. Notice the rhythm, quality, and sounds of his breathing.

RHYTHM. Breathing should be even and regular. Both sides of the chest and the abdomen should rise and fall at the same time and display equal movement on both sides.

QUALITY. Breathing should be deep. It should appear effortless and automatic.

SOUNDS. Breathing should be merely the soft swish of air as your baby inhales and exhales.

Two important signs of distress a parent can detect through observation of breathing are splinting and retraction. If there is an injury to one side of the chest—a fractured rib, for example—the child will tend to splint, or protect, that side of the chest. As a result, there will be less movement on the injured side than on the noninjured side.

Retraction occurs when air passages are narrowed or restricted—during a respiratory infection such as croup, for instance. The child is unable to take in as much air as she'd like, so she breathes more deeply and with increased vigor. This tends to create a negative pressure within the lungs that "sucks in" the softer tissues while the rib cage expands. To the observer, the muscles between the ribs and the lower end of the breastbone seem to retract inward, instead of rising upward, as the child breathes in deeply.

Both retraction and splinting should be reported promptly to the doctor.

How to Listen to Your Baby's Lung Sounds Using a Stethoscope

The most common lung ailments affecting babies and small children—things such as asthma, pneumonia, and bronchiolitis—involve excess secretions and narrowed airways within the lungs. These cause coughing, wheezing, and breathing difficul-

ties. You can detect some very distinctive abnormal sounds once you know what healthy lungs sound like.

1. Place the chest piece of your stethoscope on the right side of your baby's chest, just below the nipple. You should be able to hear very soft breath sounds in and out each time he breathes.

2. Move the chest piece around to various areas of the chest—up high, down low, around the sides. The breath sounds will be slightly different in different locations. You'll pick up the heartbeat, too, especially on the left side.

3. Now move to the back. A doctor often prefers to listen to the lungs from the back. This is partly because the breath sounds are a bit louder from the back and partly because the heartbeat is not as loud there, making it easier to hear the sounds in the left lung.

Detecting Abnormal Breathing Sounds

Unilateral Breath Sounds

Breathing sounds that seem decreased or nearly absent in one lung and exaggerated in the opposite lung are an abnormal finding that may indicate a major problem in the silent lung. Lung sounds should be about equal on both sides.

Uneven Breath Sounds

Inspiration and expiration—breathing in and breathing out, in other words—should be of approximately equal duration. A prolonged expiratory phase is a common finding in asthma and bronchiolitis.

Noisy Breathing

Noisy breathing is one of the most common breathing abnormalities. Noisy breathing can be either *chronic*—that is, long-standing—or *acute*, the kind that comes on with a cold or respiratory infection.

The chronic variety is a harmless condition that babies outgrow. One kind of chronic noisy breathing is made by the soft palate and sounds like snoring. Another form emanates lower down, in the throat. Here, the epiglottis, a little tongue of tissue that guards the entrance to the esophagus, or windpipe, vibrates when the baby breathes in. This makes a rattling, snoring noise that is more pronounced when the baby is excited and subsides markedly when she is quiet. Eventually the baby will develop better control over the soft palate or the epiglottis, and the chronic noisy breathing will disappear.

Acute noisy breathing, on the other hand, is a symptom of illness that generally accompanies a common cold. Mucus in the lower throat causes a noisy breathing or rasping sound in the chest. Such breathing has a harsh, rattling sound. It will clear up, at least temporarily, when the child coughs. If your child has this problem, encourage him to cough. If the noisy breathing clears up, it is unlikely that the child is having a serious breathing problem.

Wheezing

Wheezing and the sounds of croup are two other types of noisy breathing that can be more serious in nature. The noisy breathing of croup, a respiratory infection of the larynx, is accompanied by a very characteristic metallic or barking cough, and this may be quite frightening. (Croup and another serious illness—acute epiglottitis—are cov-

ered in Chapter 7, "How to Examine Your Baby's Nose, Throat, and Neck.") Wheezing is usually described as a whistling or musical sound in the chest. This can be heard easily through a stethoscope and often without it. Although wheezing is most commonly caused by asthma, it can also be caused by a bit of food or a small toy caught in the windpipe, as a reaction to an insect sting or some medication, or as a result of long-term illness.

There are several particularly ominous signs to watch for with wheezing. Watch the color of the child's lips. If they are bluish or dusky, this means that the blood is not receiving enough oxygen and for some reason not enough air is moving in and out of the lungs. Labored breathing is another indication of trouble, particularly if the child is unable to sleep because of this. Finally, short, quick breaths are an ominous sign. All children will breathe more rapidly if they are feverish. **But a child who is turning blue, taking short, quick breaths with difficulty, needs prompt medical attention.**

Asthma

Typical asthmatic attacks are usually triggered by some substance that the child breathes. In the spring and early summer, this substance could be pollen. Pollens blow through the air and collect on a child's body, and stick to the hair. Pollen shaken loose from a child's hair or body can often keep an attack going that might otherwise have stopped by itself.

Children with a tendency toward asthma should have a shower and shampoo every night before going to bed and should not handle pets that have been outside and might be carrying pollen on their fur. The likelihood of an asthma attack during pollen season can be reduced by keeping the child indoors on windy days and by keeping his bedroom relatively free of pollen with an air conditioner or other air-filtering device.

Other asthma triggers include house dust from house cleaning, dust mites, flowers, wood smoke, outdoor charcoal cooking, feathers, animal dander, tobacco smoke, perfumes, paints, cooking odors, and other smells or vapors. Emotional upsets can bring on an attack, and sometimes simply laughing or crying is all it will take. If the attack is severe, the child will require asthma medication. Chronic asthma should always be managed by a doctor.

Pneumonia

Pneumonia is also a serious and relatively common respiratory problem in children. Children with pneumonia often have a fever, and their breathing is shallow and labored. The only certain way to diagnose pneumonia is with a chest x-ray. If your child has a fever, acts ill, and has difficulty breathing, it is possible he has pneumonia and should be seen by a doctor.

Bronchiolitis

Bronchiolitis affects children under two, mostly in the winter months. It is potentially serious because there is widespread involvement of the small, narrow airways deep within the lungs.

The illness usually starts as a mild cold or runny nose. The infant gradually develops a heavy cough or wheezing and has difficulty breathing. Breathing becomes rapid and shallow. At this point, it is important to take the baby to a doctor.

Cystic Fibrosis

Cystic fibrosis is a genetically transmitted disease characterized by repeated lung infections. It has been estimated that 5 percent of the population carries this gene. Since it is a recessive gene, it may be passed on, unnoticed, for several generations until two individuals, each carrying the recessive gene, happen to marry. At this point, their offspring stands a one-in-four chance of inheriting cystic fibrosis.

If the child has a mild form of the disease, it may not be evident for several months or even several years. At some point, however, it becomes clear that the child is not thriving. A cough develops and hangs on; the skin tastes salty; and, most significantly, the child is not growing at the rate he should.

This is directly related to another symptom—loose, fatty stools, a sign that food is passing through the intestines without being fully digested. Consequently, the child's body is being deprived of important nutrients, vitamins and minerals. A special diet, vitamin supplements, and physical therapy to help drain the lungs of secretions are important ways to manage this disease.

Tuberculosis

Tuberculosis is often thought of as a disease of the past because public health efforts to control it have been so successful. Tuberculosis is, however, still very much with us and on the rise once again. People carrying HIV are particularly susceptible to tuberculosis, and new strains of tuberculosis germs are resistant to anti-tubercular drugs we now have. Tuberculosis is more common in crowded cities where people live in close contact with one another and are exposed to coughing by more people.

Tuberculosis may affect other parts of the body, but the most common form is tuberculosis of the lungs. In adults, the usual symptoms are a chronic cough, loss of appetite, and loss of weight. These symptoms, however, are rarely present in young children. Sometimes the only symptom in babies is persistent fever of more than two weeks' duration. The most important clue is a history of contact with someone who has the disease. If you suspect that your child may have been in contact with someone who has tuberculosis, bring this fact to the attention of your doctor. Skin testing for tuberculosis is simple and highly reliable. Treatment with specific drugs is very successful, particularly in the early stages of the disease.

Breath-Holding Spells

One of the most frustrating breathing difficulties that a parent may confront is a breath-holding spell. The usual sequence of events in a breath-holding spell is, first, a precipitating event. This event may be a minor fall, a minor injury, frustration, or simply being frightened. The child will cry, for a very short time, inhale, and then hold her breath until she becomes blue around the lips. Finally the child will pass out. At this point, the body's automatic breathing mechanism takes over. The child commences breathing and regains consciousness.

Breath-holding to the point of turning blue around the lips is extremely common. Breath-holding to the point of passing out is also fairly common. Many pediatricians will not consider a child as having a true breath-holding spell unless the child actually holds his breath long enough to lose consciousness.

Breath-holding spells usually start between the ages of six months and two years and frequently last until age four or five. Babies under six months almost never have breath-holding spells, and it is uncommon between six months and a year. If your baby is under twelve months and has a breath-holding spell that progresses to loss of consciousness, you should telephone your doctor immediately. This phenomenon is so uncommon in the younger age range that what may seem to be breath-holding is likely to be a more serious disorder.

Breath-holding spells in babies over a year are not dangerous in themselves and have nothing to do with either epilepsy or any other brain or nervous system disorder. Do not try to revive the child with mouth-to-mouth resuscitation. This is entirely unnecessary and could cause her to choke or vomit. At most, you will probably want to get an ice-cold washcloth and apply it to your child's forehead.

After the attack is over, simply go about your business. A brief hug for your child is fine, but special concern is only likely to lead to more breath-holding spells. These spells often occur when the child has a tantrum because she wants her way in some particular situation. So do not give your child anything that can be viewed as a reward after a breath-holding spell. You may be frightened by it when it happens, but try not to let her know this. Breath-holding spells usually stop by age four or five.

It is a medical emergency, of course, when a child suddenly stops breathing during illness or when there is no reason to suspect a breath-holding spell. If you think this is due to something caught in the child's trachea (windpipe), and she is choking, the emergency procedures described in Chapter 16 should be used. The emergency rescue team should be called immediately, and the child should be rushed to a hospital emergency room. Every parent should learn about the emergency procedures to follow when a child is choking. Courses are offered frequently by local hospitals and YMCAs. Take advantage of them.

Checking Vital Signs

The word *vital* means "necessary to life," and vital signs are, quite simply, signs of life. Checking vital signs is the most routine of all medical tests. Vital signs provide some of the important facts a doctor wants to know, and they are of basic importance in any health assessment. There are four vital signs:

- Pulse rate, or the number of heartbeats per minute

- Blood pressure, or the measurement of how hard the heart must work to pump blood

- Respiratory rate, or the number of breaths per minute

- Body temperature

Medical people often refer to someone's vital signs as though they were a mirror of all the systems that keep the body running. They are not the whole story, by any means, but taken together, these relatively simple statistics tell a good deal about an individual's state of health. A well-kept record of the vital signs taken at regular intervals is a valuable part of your baby's health history.

Pulse Rate

The pulse rate is the same as the heart rate. When you feel someone's pulse, you are actually feeling an artery as it momentarily swells with each heartbeat as the blood is forced through the blood vessels.

Pulses can be found behind the knees; on the inner side of the ankle just behind the large, bony prominence; on the top surface of the foot; deep in the groin area; or wherever a large artery comes near the surface of the body.

The most convenient location for taking the pulse is at the wrist. For babies younger than two years, however, listening directly to the heartbeat yields more reliable results.

How to Take the Pulse Rate of Children over Two Years

1. Find the pulse located on the inside of the wrist, below the base of the thumb. Have your child extend his hand, palm side up. You should be able to feel a groove on the inside of the wrist, bounded on the outside by a prominent wrist bone and by the cordlike tendons that are in the middle of the wrist. A large blood vessel—the radial artery—runs in this groove. With a little practice, it is easy to feel its regular pulsation.

2. Place the index and middle finger of your hand on this spot just below the base of the thumb and count the number of beats that you feel for thirty seconds. Multiply this number by two to get the beats per minute.

3. Never count the pulse rate by feeling with your thumb. There is a small artery in the thumb, and it is possible to confuse the beats from your own heart with the beats of your child's, and consequently obtain an inaccurate measurement.

How to Take the Pulse Rate of Babies Under Two Years

1. Place the chest piece of your stethoscope on the left side of your baby's chest, just below the nipple and very slightly toward the center. Lacking a stethoscope, you can hear enough through a cardboard tube from a roll of paper towels to count the heartbeat.

2. Count each lub-dub as one pulse beat.

3. Listen for thirty seconds and multiply this number by two.

The pulse rate is highest at birth and falls steadily throughout childhood. Moreover, there is a wide range of "normals" within each age group. At birth, the heart rate is approximately 130 beats per minute; by age one it is about 110; by age two, 105; and by age four, it is down to about 90 beats per minute. By adolescence, the heart rate has fallen to the normal adult rate of about 70. But changes from normal are more important than the normal itself. The only way to know your baby's normal is to find it and record it.

Take your baby's pulse rate several times to find what is normal for her. Do this when the baby is quiet. Excitement, crying, and emotional upset can elevate the pulse rate. If you are reporting a pulse rate to the doctor, indicate if the baby was crying at the time.

Other factors, such as fever or breathing difficulties, can influence the pulse rate as well. An elevated pulse rate is an additional symptom that can help confirm your suspicions of illness. At an examination during illness, tell the doctor what a normal pulse rate is for your child when he is well.

Blood Pressure

The heart pumps with a squeezing action. With each squeeze, the blood pressure rises to a peak level, and between squeezes it falls to a lower level. The highest level the blood pressure reaches is called the systolic pressure which occurs when the heart is in its squeezing phase. The lowest level the blood pressure reaches is called the diastolic pressure which occurs when the heart is refilling. Blood pressure is normally recorded as two numbers, such as 120 over 74 (120/74). The first, or larger, of the two numbers is the systolic pressure; the second, or smaller, is the diastolic pressure.

Of the four vital signs, blood pressure is the most difficult to obtain in an infant and requires special equipment. Parents are able to take their baby's blood pressure, however, and should know how. A recent series of studies indicates that hypertension, or high blood pressure, can show up in school children as young as eight. And childhood, of course, is the ideal time to acquire healthy habits in diet and exercise—two important factors in controlling high blood pressure. So keep a weather eye on your child's blood pressure.

There are two techniques for measuring blood pressure: the flush method for infants and the standard method for children over one, using a blood-pressure cuff and gauge, and a stethoscope. You can buy a blood-pressure kit in the drugstore for under thirty dollars. It is a valuable asset for the whole family.

The blood-pressure kits you can buy in a drugstore come equipped with an adult-size cuff. You will need a pediatric-size cuff, which you can obtain in a medical supply store. They come in different sizes, so choose one carefully. A cuff that is too narrow will cause a falsely elevated blood pressure reading; one that is too wide will result in a low reading. A good rule of thumb is to use a cuff that covers about two-thirds of the upper arm. For children under four, this is usually about two-and-a-half to three inches. For children between five and ten, a four-inch cuff is about right. The air bulb and pressure gauge detach easily, so you can use various size cuffs with the same bulb and gauge.

The apparatus we will describe here is the one that has a squeeze bulb and either a column of mercury or a spring dial, and requires you to listen with a stethoscope. There are more convenient (and more expensive) kinds of equipment that provide a digital readout automatically, but they are not as accurate as the equipment that requires you to squeeze and listen.

How to Take Blood Pressure of a Child over One Year

1. Wrap the cuff snugly around the upper arm, above the elbow.

2. Have the child lay his lower arm on a table, palm side up. Place the diaphragm, or flat disc, of your stethoscope in the little hollow of the elbow joint. (Remember when fitting the stethoscope to your ears to hold the earpieces so that they point slightly forward when you put on the instrument; this way they will fit snugly and comfortably into your ears.)

3. Using the squeeze bulb, pump the blood-pressure cuff up to a reading of about 120 to 140 mm on the dial. (Close the thumbscrew valve before you begin pumping.)

4. Listening carefully, crack open the air-release valve on the squeeze-bulb air pump and allow the air to escape very gradually. Listen intently as the needle begins to fall. Suddenly you will begin to hear thumping sounds. These are the sounds made by the blood as it rushes through the artery that has been partly occluded by the inflated cuff. As you continue to release air, these sounds will begin to sharply diminish and then disappear entirely.

5. Note the position of the needle on the gauge of your cuff when you first hear the sounds and also the position of the needle when the sounds disappear. The first, higher number is the systolic blood pressure; the point at which the sounds disappear is the diastolic blood pressure.

As with the pulse rate, blood pressure changes as the child grows. At one month of age, the blood pressure averages 80 systolic and 46 diastolic. The variation, however, is quite wide and systolic pressures anywhere from 65 to 95 are generally considered acceptable, with a comparable range in diastolic pressure. By one year, the systolic pressure rises to 90 or more, with the diastolic pressure rising to 55 or 60; again, there is wide variation. Record what is normal for your baby. If normal seems high to you, consult your doctor.

In babies under a year, it is difficult to obtain blood pressure using a stethoscope because of the difficulty in hearing the sounds accurately. Therefore, another measurement technique has been devised, called the flush method.

How to Take an Infant's Blood Pressure: The Flush Method

1. Wrap the pediatric-size, blood-pressure cuff around the upper arm, above the elbow.

2. Then, with your hand, firmly squeeze the lower part of the arm in order to push as much blood out of it as possible. While continuing your squeezing, pump up the blood-pressure cuff to approximately 130.

3. Release the air-bleed valve so that the pressure gradually comes down. You will notice that while the pressure in the cuff is high, the arm remains relatively light in color. Suddenly, when the pressure in the cuff is low enough, a rush of blood comes through and into the arm, and flushes to a darker color. This point, when the arm flushes darker, should be noted on the pressure dial. This is the flush blood pressure.

If you are using the flush method, you will obtain a single figure. This is the mean blood pressure. For an infant up to twelve months old, the mean blood pressure hovers around 60 to 70, but it can be as low as 50 or as high as 100. The mean blood pressure obtained using the flush method is generally about thirty points lower than the systolic figure obtained using a stethoscope.

By age three, the systolic pressure is up to about 100, with an average rise in diastolic pressure to about 65. The blood pressure then stays between 95 and 100 until the child is about eight years old. Between six and eight, the average diastolic pressure (the lower figure) may actually fall a bit to about 55. If your child's blood pressure is outside of these normal ranges, you should have it checked by the doctor.

Respiratory Rate

The respiratory rate is the number of breaths your baby takes in a minute. The respiratory rate of an infant is far higher than that of an adult. During the first year of life, the respiratory rate is approximately thirty breaths per minute. This falls off to about twenty-five per minute in the second year of life and to about twenty by age eight. At some time in the teenage years the respiratory rate drops to its normal adult rate of sixteen to eighteen breaths per minute.

How to Measure Your Baby's Respiratory Rate

1. Wait for a time when your baby is quiet and relaxed. Talking, whining, crying, and wiggling may throw off your count and increase the respiratory rate.

2. Look at your watch and count the number of times your baby's abdomen (the chest, in an older child) rises and falls for a period of thirty seconds. Multiply this number by two.

The respiratory rate is influenced not only by the condition of the lungs but also by the condition of the heart and by body temperature. An abnormally rapid respiratory rate is associated with certain kinds of lung disorders—asthma, for instance—but it is far more frequently indicative of an elevated body temperature due to illness. Record your baby's normal respiratory rate in her health record.

Body Temperature

Of the four vital signs, only body temperature remains relatively constant as your baby grows. The normal temperature, when taken by mouth, is approximately 37°C, or 98.6°F. Normal temperatures vary from one individual to another. Your child's normal temperature may be a bit higher or a bit lower.

Body temperature is generally lowest first thing in the morning, goes up gradually during the day, and peaks in the mid to late afternoon. These daily variations may be quite wide. If the body temperature is above 96°F (35°C) and below 99°F (37°C) when taken orally or below 100°F (38°C) when taken rectally, you probably have no reason to worry.

Body temperature may be measured with a mercury clinical thermometer in three ways: in the mouth, in the rectum, and under the armpit. The rectal temperature, which is the most accurate, is about a half-degree centigrade, or one degree Fahrenheit, higher than an oral reading. The axillary, or armpit, temperature (the least accurate) is about a half-degree centigrade, or one degree

Fahrenheit, lower than temperature taken in the mouth. It is important, therefore, when reporting your baby's temperature to the doctor, to tell where the temperature was taken. Do not add or subtract a degree in an attempt to make the temperature comparable to an oral reading. This may only confuse the doctor. Simply report the numbers and the location.

There are patches you can stick on the baby's forehead that produce a temperature reading or a color change, but these are quite inaccurate. There is also a gadget you can stick in the ear that produces a digital readout on a little screen. This, too, is inaccurate since you frequently don't fit it snugly enough in the ear to produce a good reading. As of now, the old clinical thermometer is still the best way to go.

Taking your baby's body temperature and interpreting your findings are covered in detail in Chapter 13. Don't wait until your baby is sick, however, to find out what his normal body temperature is. Take this measurement several times while he is well, and record the average figure in your baby's personal health record. This will give you a valuable basis for comparison later if you suspect your baby is sick.

CHAPTER 4

HOW TO OBSERVE, EXAMINE, AND DEAL WITH YOUR BABY'S DIGESTIVE SYSTEM

Long before the limbs take shape in the womb, before the embryo tail disappears, before the features of the face are etched, a baby's digestive system has begun to take form. The cells of the embryo group themselves along three longitudinal structures. One of these, called the notochord, is destined to become the backbone. The other two are simple tubes, one of which develops into the spinal cord and brain and the other into the digestive system.

As the fetus develops, this primitive digestive tube acquires new characteristics. Here it swells into the stomach; there it lengthens to form the intestines, coiling up neatly within the abdominal cavity. Nerve endings that will one day trigger peristaltic waves, which propel food along its length, line the inner surfaces. And other food-processing organs—the liver and pancreas—sprout budlike from the walls of the developing tube.

Shortly before birth, baby's digestive system undergoes a final spurt of development. At the same time, the baby has been practicing sucking and swallowing skills, sucking his thumb while still in the womb. The result, at birth, is a highly efficient process called digestion that takes in food at one end, extracts the nutrients, and excretes what it can't use at the other end.

Problems with digestive function range from a simple refusal to eat certain foods to disorders that are painful or complicated and sometimes even life-threatening. Parents are often concerned about digestive function because a great deal of attention is focused on food intake and bowel movements. This is entirely appropriate because, unless adequate nutrition is available, children do not grow and develop normally.

How the Digestive Process Works

Despite the seeming complexity of the mysterious process that goes on deep inside your baby's body, the process of digestion is, in essence, simply a predictable journey down a winding tube, with predictable events occurring along the way. Once you recognize this, it's easy to visualize the various

45

structures that make up the digestive system and the way they work.

The digestive process starts in the mouth, where the mucuslike saliva makes the food slippery for easier swallowing and begins to break down food into elements the body can use. Chewing plays an important role in digestion here. Unless food is thoroughly broken up into small particles, the stomach and small intestine have great difficulty in digesting it.

From the mouth, the food proceeds down the esophagus, which is a flexible tube that runs just behind the windpipe and into the stomach. During the act of swallowing, a small structure in the back of the throat, called the epiglottis, closes over the windpipe to prevent food from going into the lungs instead of to the stomach. Occasionally the epiglottis doesn't quite make it in time, and small amounts of milk or other fluids enter the trachea, setting off a violent spasm of coughing—what we call "food going down the wrong pipe."

At about the end of the breastbone, the esophagus portion of the digestive tube widens into a baglike enlargement, which is the stomach. A valve at the entrance to the stomach keeps food in the stomach from reentering the esophagus. Compared to an adult's J-shaped stomach, an infant's stomach is round and, of course, considerably smaller.

The stomach secretes hydrochloric acid, which helps break up food into very small, easily digested pieces. Fortunately, the lining of the stomach is highly resistant to acid. A certain amount of digestion occurs in the stomach, but contrary to popular belief, very little absorption takes place here. (*Digestion* is the breaking up and processing of food; *absorption* is the transport of nutrients from the digestive tract into the bloodstream.)

The food particles then are squirted through a second valve into the small intestine. The adjective *small*, in this case, refers to the diameter of the tube, not to its length. If stretched out, the small and large intestines together would measure six times the body's length—about thirty feet long in an adult.

The small intestine is conventionally divided into three segments: the relatively short first segment is called the duodenum; the longest, middle segment, is called the jejunum; and the last segment is called the ileum. Important action takes place in the duodenum. The intestinal wall secretes its own digestive enzymes and the pancreas, which lies just below the stomach and slightly to the left of midline, adds its very important enzymes. The duodenum loops under the pancreas, and a little tube or duct runs from the head of the pancreas into the duodenum. Whenever the body senses food coming into the duodenum, the pancreas is stimulated to produce digestive enzymes, which come pouring into the duodenum through this duct.

This is also where the liver enters the digestive picture. The liver is a large organ that lies up against the diaphragm. Its contribution to digestion is the production of a yellowish substance called bile, which is stored in the gallbladder until needed. The bile duct from the liver through the gallbladder enters the small intestine right next to the duct from the pancreas. When the body senses that food is in the small intestine, particularly fatty food, the flow of bile is stimulated; that is, the gallbladder squeezes down and the bile is delivered into the duodenum.

As food moves down the small bowel, it is gradually digested, and anything of nutritive value is absorbed. The body is quite selective and has special mechanisms for absorbing each substance. Food nutrients are absorbed into the bloodstream through millions of fingerlike structures called

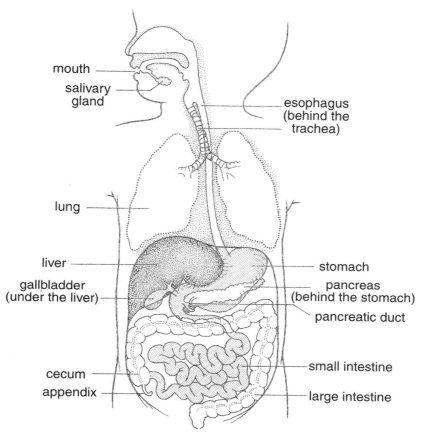

The digestive system

villi. The nutrients are then transported by a special set of blood vessels called the portal circulation to the liver for final processing. Here, the food nutrients are transformed into the actual substances the body can use for energy, growth, and repair. This central biochemical function explains the large size of the liver and stresses its importance in all metabolic processes.

The small intestine finally ends in the lower right quarter of the abdomen, where it joins the large intestine, the last section of the digestive tube. Here again, the adjective *large* refers to the diameter of the tube in this section, not to its length. It is actually much shorter than the small

intestine. A short "pouch," called the cecum, marks the spot where the small intestine joins the large intestine. From this pouch, extending downward, is a wormlike structure—the appendix—which has no digestive function.

From its beginning in the right lower quadrant, the large bowel travels upward, then across the top of the abdomen to the left upper quadrant, and finally down and inward to its end at the anal opening.

The main function of the large bowel is the concentration and storage of nonabsorbable waste matter. As waste matter moves along, it is concentrated from a watery slurry into solid fecal matter, which is finally excreted through the anus as a bowel movement. This concentration is largely a matter of the packing of material, and the absorption of water.

The large intestine contains large numbers of friendly bacteria that help keep the intestines free of harmful bacteria. The friendly bacteria also help to maintain normal function within the large bowel. If, because of illness or prolonged antibiotic treatment, the friendly bacterial colonies are disturbed or partially eradicated, inflammation may occur as harmful bacteria invade the large intestine. It is important to reestablish these colonies in order to regain normal bowel function.

How to Examine Your Baby's Abdomen

Examining your baby's abdomen begins with some simple observations, followed by listening to and finally feeling, or palpating, the abdomen.

1. *Inspect.* If your baby is standing, or is held upright, the abdomen is well-rounded and protruding, giving him a potbellied appearance. This is normal and persists up to about age three, when the abdomen begins to flatten out. The skin should be smooth and taut.

   Observe the bellybutton (the umbilicus or navel). This is usually somewhat sunken, but some babies have bellybuttons that protrude just a bit— maybe a quarter of an inch—and this is perfectly normal. Some babies have a minor defect between the muscles of the abdominal wall in the area of the umbilicus that allows a loop of small intestine to push up and create a lump in that area from time to time. This lump usually becomes more evident when the baby cries, subsiding almost entirely

when the baby is asleep. This is an umbilical hernia. These hernias rarely cause any problem. Treatment with straps or adhesive tape is not effective and may even be harmful. Small hernias of this type usually disappear spontaneously by one year of age. Larger umbilical hernias may persist longer, but even these generally close up by themselves. Surgery, if necessary, is not advised until age three to five years.

Hernias can turn up elsewhere on the abdominal wall. A femoral hernia, seen more frequently in girls, shows up as a small mass or lump in the area where the thigh joins the abdomen. An inguinal hernia, more common in boys, can show itself as a swelling in the groin, or as a piece of bowel that has slipped into the scrotum. (This is described in more detail in Chapter 11, "Checking on Baby's Bottom and Urinary System.") Any masses you observe on the abdomen should be called to the doctor's attention.

2. *Listen.* Place the round diaphragm of your stethoscope anywhere on your baby's abdomen. Listen, and you will hear bowel sounds. This is a gurgling noise made by the slurry of food as it is pushed through the small intestine. Normal bowel sounds are typically heard every ten to fifteen seconds. But if your baby has not eaten recently, bowel sounds may be less noticeable. You can often stimulate them by stroking the abdomen with the back of your fingernail. The absence of all bowel sounds in a child who also has other signs of illness is a serious finding and may indicate an intestinal blockage. Bowel sounds may be very quiet at times, however, so before you conclude there are none, you must listen for several minutes by the clock.

3. *Palpate.* The last step in examining the abdomen is palpation, a technique of pressing and feeling with the fingers. Palpate in all four quadrants of the abdomen. A quadrant is simply a quarter of the abdomen—baby's top right, top left, lower right, and lower left. The umbilicus is the center point. (Do not include the chest, of course, when you think of quadrants of the abdomen.)

Be sure baby is calm and relaxed. Place your hand on the baby's stomach and, using gentle to moderate pressure, push the flats of your fingers inward. Do this carefully in all four quadrants. You will probably not feel anything because the small intestines that fill most of the abdominal cavity slip easily out of the way. But sometimes, if the child is particularly constipated, it is possible to feel a long, sausage-like mass on the left side. This is the large intestine, filled with feces.

If severe pain has sent the abdominal muscles into spasm, the entire abdominal area will feel tense and hard (and your baby will be screaming). Barring these exceptions, however, the abdomen should feel soft, and your gentle palpation should not cause distress. Anything else should be reported to your doctor.

Bowel Movements

Normal bowel movements in a baby vary a good deal with age and diet, and from one individual to another. Stomach capacity is small in a newborn, and food moves quickly through the digestive tract. This means more frequent bowel movements in the very young infant. Three to five stools per day by the end of the first week are typical. But it is not unusual for an infant to have as many as six or seven movements a day, or fewer than three. As stomach capacity increases and the digestive system matures, food is processed at a more leisurely pace, and bowel movements eventually decrease to one a day, or even to one every two or three days. Breast-fed babies, in particular, may go without a bowel movement for a few days.

Since disturbances of the intestinal tract and other illnesses tend to have an effect on the character of bowel movements, you should be able to recognize what is normal at a given age for your child.

Recognizing Normal Infant Bowel Movements

A newborn infant usually passes the first stools within twenty-four hours. This first movement is a sticky, greenish gray and consists of debris that has accumulated in the digestive tube before birth. It is called meconium. Passage of meconium confirms that the digestive tube is functioning. By the second or third day, these meconium stools will gradually be replaced with greenish brown stools that may contain some milk curds. These are referred to as transitional stools.

Once feeding is well established, the stools become yellow to golden in color, with the consistency of thick cream sauce. These are typical milk stools. Breast-fed babies will have somewhat softer stools, while babies receiving a cow's milk formula will have somewhat firmer stools, with a more offensive odor.

Diarrhea

Diarrhea is commonly defined as a sudden increase in the frequency and looseness of bowel movements. It's hard, however, to say precisely how many movements of exactly what consistency constitute diarrhea. Infants and breast-fed babies normally have softer stools than bottle-fed babies and older children. Furthermore, bowel movements vary widely from one infant to another. One baby may pass a single, firm stool every other day, whereas another may normally have a half-dozen small, loose stools daily. Far more important than a definition, then, in recognizing diarrhea is a comparison with what parents know is normal bowel function for their baby.

How to Recognize Diarrhea

Three kinds of changes in your baby's normal pattern of bowel movements should enable you to recognize diarrhea; they are:

1. A sudden, noticeable increase in the number of bowel movements

2. A noticeable increase in the fluid content—that is, loose, watery stools

3. A greenish tinge in the color of the stools (which may not be apparent in mild cases)

Assessing Diarrhea

Diarrhea can have any number of causes—a "bug" going around or sensitivity to a certain food are two of the more common culprits. In mild cases, diarrhea may be the only obvious indicator of illness. Mild diarrhea can be managed at home. Moderate and more severe cases will require professional supervision. Upon determining that your baby has diarrhea, your first consideration should be deciding how bad a case you are dealing with and then noticing if there are other symptoms of distress as well.

MILD DIARRHEA. The stools increase in frequency from what you know is normal for your baby. They are softer and mushier than usual. There are no other signs of illness or distress.

DIARRHEA WITH OTHER SYMPTOMS. In addition to more frequent and softer stools, notice if there are other signs of illness or distress: fever, vomiting, pain, lethargy (the baby looks and acts sick). Any combination of other symptoms with diarrhea in a child under one year should be brought to the doctor's attention. A combination of diarrhea and vomiting can lead very quickly to dehydration.

SEVERE DIARRHEA. Severe diarrhea, which warrants bringing your baby to medical attention, is more than one episode an hour at any age and even a single episode per hour for a baby under one year. Severe diarrhea combined with other symptoms is enough reason to go to the doctor. Blood in a diarrhea stool is also reason to call your doctor at once.

Dealing with Mild Diarrhea

If the diarrhea is mild, and your child does not appear to be ill otherwise, there are a few things you can try. But if diarrhea persists for more than a day or two, consult the doctor.

Keep in mind that diarrhea stools are very irritating to baby's skin, so take extra care to protect the skin in the diaper area. Change soiled diapers promptly and apply a film of a soothing baby cream or lotion after cleansing.

IN BREAST-FED INFANTS. Breast-fed babies rarely develop serious diarrhea, and breast-feeding should not be stopped for mild diarrhea. The only thing the baby may need is extra water. Offer the baby a supplemental bottle containing only water between feedings. If the diarrhea persists beyond a day or two, be sure to call your doctor.

IN BOTTLE-FED INFANTS. Bottle-fed babies should be taken off formula entirely and given only clear liquids for twenty-four hours. Among the clear liquids you can use are commercial drinks containing electrolytes that are available from your pharmacy without prescription; ask your pharmacist for recommendations. Diluted fruit juices, weak broth, or gelatin water are helpful. Gelatin water is made by adding one package of flavored gelatin to a quart of water, or twice as much water as you'd usually use, in order to dilute the sugar content. Kool-Aid, ginger ale, cola, and sodas are all poor choices for the treatment of diarrhea because of their high sugar content, which will simply aggravate the already disturbed bowel. Fruit drinks that are mostly sugar and only 10 percent fruit juice should also be avoided. Read the labels before using fruit drinks.

After twenty-four hours of clear liquids, if the baby has been using a cow's milk formula, ask your doctor about starting your baby on a soy milk formula. Soy formulas tend to be less irritating to the bowel than cow's milk formulas. For the first twenty-four hours, use half-strength formula, then use regular-strength soy formula for about one week.

If your baby is eating solids, you may wish to try rice cereal, applesauce, strained bananas, or strained carrots. Do not give other solids during this week because they may be irritating.

If mild diarrhea persists for more than three or four days, be sure to call your doctor.

IN OLDER BABIES (SIX MONTHS TO TWO YEARS). If your baby is older than six months,

diarrhea should be treated by immediately stopping milk, ice cream, and other milk products. If you are still breast-feeding, call your doctor for advice. It is important that the child receive adequate fluids, and those stated previously will be quite satisfactory. Avoid giving high sugar-containing fluids since they may contribute to the problem.

After a day or two of clear liquids, a few solid foods can be reintroduced (if your baby has already graduated to table foods). On the first day, limit the child to crackers, toast, bland soups, applesauce, and rice. On the second day, soft-boiled eggs, noodles, and lean meats may be added. Chicken and turkey are preferable to beef. On the third day, cottage cheese, yogurt, and soft-cooked fruits may be added. By the fourth day, you might wish to try adding cooked vegetables to return the child to a regular diet.

IN YOUNG CHILDREN (TWO YEARS AND UP). For children over two years, the same approach should be used as for those under two, with the exception that the progression to a normal diet may be a bit faster. After the first day, raw fruits and vegetables, beans, and spices should be avoided. But otherwise, a relatively normal bland diet can be taken. Eliminate milk products and ice cream from the diet as long as any diarrhea is present. After the diarrhea has been entirely cleared for twenty-four hours, a normal diet can be resumed.

If the diarrhea becomes more severe or does not improve in forty-eight hours on the diets suggested, call your doctor.

How to Recognize Dehydration

Considerable water is lost during bouts of diarrhea. This is the real threat that diarrhea poses to a baby—water loss and the dehydration that follows.

Dehydration rapidly leads to shock and can be fatal in infants and small children. Your prime concern, then, while treating a baby for diarrhea is watching for symptoms of dehydration.

1. Lack of urination for over eight hours in a baby under one year or for more than twelve hours in a child over one year suggests dehydration.

2. The inside of your baby's mouth should feel moist and wet, like your own. A dry mouth and tongue are signs of dehydration.

3. Gently pinch the skin of your baby's abdomen between your thumb and forefinger. Normal skin is elastic and will snap back almost instantly. In a dehydrated baby, however, the skin develops a doughy consistency—when you pinch it, it will stay heaped up almost like putty for a few seconds.

4. Poor skin color—pale to grayish—is another indicator of dehydration.

Constipation

At the other end of the scale from diarrhea is constipation, in which bowel movements are hard, infrequent, and painful to pass. Just as a diagnosis of diarrhea is based on a comparison with the child's normal pattern of bowel movements, constipation is also an individual matter.

The more common pattern for bowel movements in children past infancy is one per day, but some children normally have two or even three bowel movements a day, and some perfectly normal children go as long as three days without a movement. After the second month of life, many breast-fed babies will have perfectly normal, soft bowel movements quite infrequently.

The important thing to note about frequency of bowel movements is the normal pattern for the individual child. If your child generally has been having bowel movements on a daily basis, going for a period of three days without a movement could certainly be considered constipation. If your child only has a bowel movement once every other day, though, you wouldn't consider him constipated unless he has had no bowel movement for four days.

Occasionally, a child unwittingly brings on constipation by holding back or retaining his bowel movements. Sometimes the underlying cause is a break in the skin in the anal area. Even a tiny break can be very painful, and the child tends to hold his stools, putting off having a bowel movement. Consequently, the fecal material inside the rectum becomes dryer and harder and increasingly difficult to pass. Soon your child has a self-perpetuating case of constipation. Have a doctor verify and treat this situation.

Another kind of stool retention sometimes shows up in the early stages of toilet training, but it also can happen later in children as old as eight years. During this first stage of independence when a child is saying "no" right and left, his nay-saying may carry over into the bathroom. In response to your urgent entreaties to use the toilet, he will refuse to go at all. This pattern has been called psychologic stool-holding because there is no physical reason for the child's behavior. If this pattern is allowed to persist for months or even years, correction becomes more difficult than if measures are taken within the first few months. Consult the doctor about this.

Finally, observe whether your child is soiling himself with small amounts of relatively loose stool. If this is the case, he may have a large, very hard mass of stool in his rectum, and you should seek medical advice about the best way of getting it out.

If your child has gone several days without a bowel movement but has the sensation of wanting to have one, several home remedies can be tried. Sometimes simply having your child sit in a warm bathtub and relax will do the trick. If this doesn't help, ask your doctor about inserting a glycerine suppository to stimulate the lower bowel into action. If both of these remedies fail and if your child does not have abdominal pain, fever, or other symptoms of illness, the doctor may recommend an enema. **But be sure to get the doctor's say-so before going ahead with this.**

How to Give an Enema

Before giving an enema to a child, tell her—simply and briefly—what you are going to do and what will happen. You will need a combination water bottle with a hose and a pediatric enema tip.

1. Do not use the commercial enema solutions available in the drugstore for adults. These are intended for use with adults, and their ingredients are too harsh for children. Instead, ask your pharmacist for a preparation for children, or prepare your own solution of a level teaspoon of table salt and a pint of lukewarm tap water. If the temperature of the enema water feels too warm on your hand, it is clearly too warm for the bowel.

2. Measure the proper amount of salt solution into the water bottle: for a baby nine to twelve months old, use four ounces; one to three years of age, six ounces; three to six years of age, eight ounces. Do not put more solution than you will use into the enema bag.

3. Place a large towel on the bathroom floor for your child to lie on. Position the child on her left side, with her right leg pulled up and the left leg straightened so that she will be partly rolled forward on her stomach. Lubricate the enema tip with a little petroleum jelly and insert it one-and-a-half to two inches into the rectum. It should slide in easily. **Do not force it or you may do damage to the bowel wall.**

4. Holding the enema bag not more than two feet above the level of the child's anus, allow the solution to run in gradually. Encourage the child to retain the solution as long as she can, hopefully for two to three minutes. Rubbing the child's back gently sometimes helps. Infants and young children, of course, are not capable of holding the solution in the rectum after it is administered, so you should hold the buttocks together for a minute or two to allow the solution a chance to work.

5. When the child expels the enema solution, the stool matter will be expelled with it. An older child may make it to the toilet in time. But don't scold a child for using the towel. That's what it's there for.

Preventing Constipation

The best approach to the long-term treatment of constipation is dietary. Adding sugar to the diet of a bottle-fed baby helps. Add a tablespoon of corn syrup in each bottle for a few days. Adding strained apricots and prunes (or prune juice) to the diet will also be helpful.

For older children, increasing the amount of bran in their diet is probably the simplest measure. Serve bran cereal for breakfast. Or stir a half-teaspoon of plain, unmilled bran (available by the jar in many grocery stores) into applesauce or orange juice. Other natural cereals are a good source of fiber. Lower on the list but still effective are shredded wheat, oatmeal, graham crackers, and whole wheat bread. Fruits and vegetables help. Prunes, figs, and dates have a wide reputation for effectiveness. Celery, lettuce, carrots, and leafy vegetables are also helpful in providing bulk, particularly if they are eaten several times a day. All of these foods are more effective raw than cooked.

Spitting Up, Vomiting, and Other Varieties of Stomach Return

In infants, the muscular valve between the esophagus and the stomach—the cardiac sphincter—is relatively weak, making it easy for small amounts of food to be forced back up the esophagus and out the mouth again. This is a common occurrence after feedings and does not mean that anything is wrong.

More forceful return of stomach contents, of course, is another thing. Four terms are used by doctors to distinguish the various degrees of this common complaint. Recognizing the differences among them is an important first step in determining if something is wrong.

SPITTING UP. Food that dribbles out of an infant's mouth soon after feeding is referred to as spitting up.

REGURGITATION. Regurgitation refers to the return of undigested food from the stomach, the kind that sometimes comes with burping.

VOMITING. Vomiting is a more forceful return of stomach contents and may be accompanied by nausea in an older child.

PROJECTILE VOMITING. Projectile vomiting is readily recognized by the force with which stomach contents are propelled from the mouth. The vomitus may be ejected as much as two to four feet away if the child is lying on his side, or as high as a foot if the baby is lying on his back.

Spitting Up and Regurgitation

Of the four degrees of stomach return, spitting up and regurgitation are quite normal in young infants. Some babies have a harder time keeping food down than others and habitually regurgitate some food after each feeding. The problem is often associated with a weak, or relaxed, cardiac sphincter. When the cardiac sphincter is not snug enough to keep food in the stomach, some of the food escapes back up the esophagus and out the mouth. This usually corrects itself as baby's digestive apparatus matures. Until it does, there are some easy measures you can take to control the symptoms.

How to Deal with Spitting Up and Regurgitation in Infants

If your baby has a tendency to spit up, try modifying your feeding procedure as follows:

1. Keep the baby in a sitting position during feeding and for a while afterward.

2. Burp her frequently during feedings.

3. Consult your doctor about trying a slightly thickened diet, such as adding a bit of infant cereal to feeding.

Vomiting

Occasional attacks of vomiting are so common in infants and small children that they can almost be considered a normal part of life. An infant's digestive tract is still immature, and any number of things can upset it. Simple overfeeding sometimes causes breast-fed babies to vomit. If your baby has vomited only once or twice and seems otherwise quite normal, you should try limiting the time your baby nurses on each breast.

A flu bug or other virus that upsets the digestive tract is a common cause of vomiting. In addition, food allergies can frequently result in vomiting, and intestinal obstructions—less common but very serious—will also induce vomiting. Even something that seems unrelated, such as a head injury that irritates the brain, can be the underlying cause, since the act of vomiting is actually initiated by the central nervous system.

Keep in mind that vomiting in itself is not an illness—it is merely a symptom of illness. Furthermore, it is not the act of vomiting, but the consequence of it, that may pose a threat to your child. More important than food loss is the fluid lost through vomiting; and when vomiting is combined with diarrhea—both common flu symptoms—the resulting water loss can be deadly. So, do not allow a baby under six months to vomit repeatedly for more than six hours or a child over six months to vomit repeatedly for more than twelve hours before taking him to the doctor.

Call the doctor immediately if vomiting is associated with any of the following symptoms:

1. Vomiting that contains blood

2. Vomiting that contains green bile

3. Vomiting accompanied by diarrhea

4. Vomiting associated with high fever

5. Vomiting with abdominal pain that has lasted more than two hours

6. Vomiting without abdominal pain that has been going on continuously for more than six hours in a baby younger than six months or more than twelve hours in a child over six months

7. Vomiting associated with stupor, confusion, and/or the inability of the child to touch his chin to the center of his chest

8. Projectile vomiting

Some parents are quick to call the doctor whenever their child begins to vomit in the hope that the physician will prescribe a medicine that will halt the vomiting and spare the child the discomfort of this unpleasant process. Although some very good drugs have been developed for the control of vomiting, none of them have been shown to be effective in stopping the usual childhood vomiting and in themselves may have dangerous or unpleasant side effects.

How to Deal with Mild Vomiting

If the vomiting is mild and sporadic, and if your child does not show any of the associated danger signs listed above, simple home remedies may be tried for up to forty-eight hours.

1. Keep the child's stomach relatively empty, avoiding all solid foods for at least twelve hours; nothing at all need be given for the first six hours. After that, clear fluids—those you can see through—may be given in very small quantities. Good choices are cola, ginger ale, or Seven Up, which has been stirred or shaken so that no bubbles remain. Start with a teaspoonful every fifteen to twenty minutes. If this is tolerated, try a tablespoonful. You may double the total amount each hour as long as the child tolerates it. If he vomits

again, rest the stomach completely for one to two hours and then start over with smaller amounts.

2. Another good remedy is cola syrup. One to two teaspoons, depending on age, every twenty to thirty minutes, may help settle the stomach before you begin clear fluids.

3. After about eight hours with no episodes of vomiting, solid foods may be gradually re-introduced. For babies, start with foods like applesauce and cereals; for older children, toast and bland soups are usually best. Children who are otherwise healthy can easily go without food for two days without harmful effects. But fluids are another matter. Remember, vomiting children are likely to become dehydrated, and it is important that a certain amount of fluids be provided. A common error, though, is to give too much fluid too quickly. Never give your child as much as he wants to drink. This will almost certainly lead to further vomiting, and the child will vomit up more fluid than he took in, amounting to a net loss. Offering fluids in a small glass, such as a shot glass, gives the child some control and still limits the amount taken at one swallow.

4. Finally, if your child is taking an essential medicine, such as an anticonvulsant and is vomiting up the medicine, you should contact your physician immediately for instructions.

Swallowed Objects

It's not hard to visualize the path and ultimate destination of a swallowed object. More often than not, what goes in one end will come out the other. Consider, for example, the fate of two or three plastic beads swallowed by a child. The body is unable to convert the plastic into an absorbable form, and it is also unable to break up the beads into the small pieces necessary for digestion to take place. Consequently the objects spend a day or two traveling through the intestinal tract, coming out eventually with a splash in the middle of a bowel movement.

Most swallowed objects—including marbles, coins, beads, buttons, and fruit pits—pass easily through the system. If you turn around just in time to see your child gulp and grin, and you don't know what went down, observe her reaction. If your baby does not cough, wheeze, cry, rub her throat, or otherwise show signs of distress, the object is no doubt safely launched on its journey. Watch the bowel movements for a few days to reassure yourself that the object has passed through.

When to Worry About a Swallowed Object

Not all swallowed objects are harmless, of course, and you should take immediate action in response to any of the following circumstances:

LONG AND SHARP OBJECTS. Items such as straight pins, hair pins, bones, needles, and large safety pins present a potential danger since they can become lodged in one of the many twists and turns of the digestive tube. If you believe your child has swallowed a long, sharp object, you should consult your doctor even though the doctor may do nothing except take an x-ray and watch the child. Even relatively large, threatening objects often pass through the entire intestinal tract without causing any trouble at all.

OBJECTS LODGED IN THE ESOPHAGUS. If the object seems to be stuck in the esophagus, giving your child some dry bread to eat may help move things along. A lump of dry bread going down the esophagus will often pull a coin or other small object along with it into the stomach. If this doesn't work, see the doctor promptly.

Large objects can become lodged in the lower part of the esophagus just before it enters the stomach and refuse to go further. If left there they can erode the wall of the esophagus and lead to very serious consequences.

TOXIC OBJECTS. Small alkaline batteries are potentially dangerous because if they leak they may burn the lining of the digestive tract. If you believe that your baby has swallowed a battery or other toxic object, consult the doctor without delay.

AN OBJECT LODGED IN THE AIRWAY. A foreign object can also be breathed into the airway. Nuts, seeds, and popcorn are common offenders here. If your child begins gagging, wheezing, or coughing, he has probably breathed in a foreign object. Even if the first coughing fit subsides, take the child to the doctor anyway. If the object has entered the lung, it can cause a respiratory infection.

Choking, in which the object blocks the airway, is a true medical emergency. The child who is choking cannot speak, cannot cough, turns blue, and collapses. Learn how to deal with choking in Chapter 16, "How to Recognize and Deal with Medical Emergencies." Read it now. When there is a need to know, there won't be time to learn.

POISONOUS MATERIAL. If your child swallows cleaning agents or other chemicals, medicines, poisonous plants, or the like, it is a medical emergency.

See Chapter 16, "How to Recognize and Deal with Medical Emergencies."

Never try to make your child vomit in the hope of retrieving a swallowed object. It will do more harm than good.

Recognizing Liver Disorders

You will recall that the liver produces bile, the yellowish substance important in the digestion of fats. When the liver is not functioning properly, bile can back up in the bile ducts and circulate to parts of the body where it normally wouldn't go, producing a yellowing effect on the skin, the nails, and the whites of the eyes. This effect is known as jaundice, and it is a symptom of liver problems, not a disease in itself.

The mild jaundice of the newborn, discussed in Chapter 1, is a normal occurrence that usually sets in within the first week of life and clears up by itself shortly thereafter. Jaundice in an older baby, however, is most likely caused by hepatitis, an inflammation of the liver. There are several varieties of hepatitis, each caused by a different virus—hepatitis A, B, or C.

Hepatitis A is spread among people, usually by ingesting fecally contaminated food or water, so it is liable to be encountered in places where many people are involved in food handling and where hand washing is not done as scrupulously as it should be. Restaurants and day-care centers are often among the offenders. If your child is in day care with large numbers of children or if you are traveling with your child in developing countries, talk to your doctor about immunization. The upside of hepatitis A is that while it can make a child quite ill, the cure rate and recovery is nearly 100 percent.

Hepatitis B and C, however, can lead to chronic liver disease. These viruses are passed along via body fluids—blood, saliva, sexual intercourse, and, among intravenous drug users, by exchanging dirty needles. Immunization against hepatitis B has joined the battery of childhood immunizations among most pediatricians. Ask your doctor.

If your child develops hepatitis, she will typically lose all appetite, tire easily, feel nauseated, vomit, run a slight fever, and act lethargic—all common flu symptoms. A tip-off that suggests hepatitis is tenderness in the upper right abdomen, where the liver is located.

Only after this first phase, which lasts about a week, will evidence of jaundice become noticeable. The urine will darken, the stools will become lighter in color, and the skin will be tinged with yellow. Any evidence of jaundice should be called to the doctor's attention. Because hepatitis is contagious, watch other members of the family for signs of illness.

Failure to Thrive

Remember that the basic function of the digestive system is to bring nutrients into the body where they can be used for growth and development and for the energy to run and play. If your child is not gaining weight and is not growing properly—in short, failing to thrive—he may have a disorder affecting food absorption even though his bowel movements appear relatively normal to you, he is not vomiting, and he has a good appetite.

Children with food absorption disorders sometimes develop the potbellied look of malnutrition. They tend to rank below the third percentile on the National Center for Health Statistics (NCHS) growth charts in Chapter 14. If you see this con-

dition developing, yet you know your child is receiving a good, nutritious diet, you should bring this to the attention of your doctor.

Colic

Colic is abdominal pain experienced by very young babies, usually up to the age of three or four months, though it can continue a bit longer. Typically, a half hour after an afternoon or evening feeding, baby goes into a "colic pose" by drawing the legs up to the abdomen. And the baby screams. The screaming may go on for hours despite anything you do to comfort the baby, and it is this continuous screaming that parents of colicky babies never forget.

In spite of the obvious discomfort, colicky babies thrive, gain weight, and are entirely well otherwise. You'll want to check with your doctor to be sure the pain and crying are due to colic, but once that diagnosis is made, you have to make up your mind to live with it until the episodes stop by themselves after three or four months.

How to Handle a Colicky Baby

Doctors recommend various things to try to relieve colic (and there is no end of advice from mothers of ex-colicky babies), but if your baby is colicky, chances are he will continue to be colicky until it goes away by itself. Here are some things to try:

1. Apply warmth to the baby's abdomen in the form of a well-covered hot water bottle or a well-covered heating pad.

2. Burp the baby during and after feedings.

3. Try smaller, more frequent feedings.

4. Comfort the baby and try to maintain as calm and stable an environment as possible.

Parents often need more treatment in the presence of a colicky baby than the baby does. The continuous crying and the sense of helplessness it inspires in parents can severely jeopardize the baby–parent relationship. Here are some things parents can do to survive the colicky period:

- Accept the colic for what it is. Don't blame yourself as a bad parent. And don't blame the baby. It is a legitimate ailment, and the baby is neither "bad" nor "spoiled." These are false and harmful reasons often given to explain colic.

- Whenever possible, mother and father should take turns comforting the baby. Call upon grandparents and understanding friends to give you relief. Get out of the house for some free time.

- Don't be afraid to talk about negative feelings you may have that are inspired by the constant crying. If the episodes of colic leave you severely depressed or angry, consider talking it out with a mental health specialist.

For more about colic, refer to Chapter 13, "How Can I Tell if My Baby Is Sick?"

CHAPTER 5

HOW TO TEST YOUR BABY'S EARS AND HEARING

The ability to hear is one of your baby's most vital links with the world, and even newborn babies learn to sort out the countless sounds of the world around them. Scientists have found that babies as young as three or four weeks old can distinguish between their mothers' voices and those of strangers.

The formation of language sounds depends on a child's ability to imitate sounds she hears others making. What she doesn't hear, she can't imitate. A hearing problem, then, interferes with both listening and speaking. So the earlier a hearing loss can be detected, the sooner a child can begin learning how to compensate for this handicap.

The Anatomy of the Ear

Before you examine your baby's ears and check for hearing, it is helpful to understand how the ear is constructed and how it works. The ear is divided into three sections: the outer or external ear, the middle ear, and the inner ear.

The Outer Ear

The outer ear consists of the familiar, shell-like structure that is as much of the ear as can be seen without a special instrument. The outer ear acts as a funnel, catching sounds and channeling them into the external auditory canal. This canal runs a little less than an inch inside the head and is sealed off at its inner end by a membrane called the eardrum. You should be able to see the eardrum using an otoscope (after a demonstration by your doctor and following the instructions given later in this chapter). The eardrum is as far as you can see since it obstructs any view of the middle and inner ear.

The Middle Ear

The middle ear consists of a chamber containing three miniscule bones that transmit sounds from the eardrum to the inner ear. Because the middle ear is sealed in by the eardrum, changes in air pressure around us would be painful and even destructive if this cavity did not have some other

61

connection to the outside world. This connection is provided by the Eustachian tube, which goes from the middle ear to the back of the throat. Its function is to equalize pressure on both sides of the eardrum.

When pressure on the outside of the eardrum changes for some reason—a loud noise, a change in atmospheric pressure, or a ride in an elevator— the pressure in the middle ear must adjust to the change. If pressure equalization does not occur, we say that our ears feel plugged, and we cannot hear properly until they are unplugged. Most of us have experienced this feeling when flying or driving in the mountains. In order to unplug our ears in these situations, we swallow or yawn. This action opens the Eustachian tubes in the throat, thereby providing the middle ear with access to the outside and a means of regulating air pressure on both sides of the drum.

The Eustachian tube is a bit shorter and straighter in small children than in adults, so bacteria have an easier time getting from the throat to the middle ear. This is why young children, as a rule, have more ear problems than older children and adults.

The Inner Ear

The inner ear is entirely encased in bone and contains the cochlea and the semicircular canals. The cochlea, a tiny structure with the shape of a snail's shell, transmits sounds to the brain via the auditory nerve. The brain decodes the sounds and converts them into meaningful messages.

The fluid-filled semicircular canals are responsible for a vital function that has to do with position sense. Vestibular function, as this capability is called, is one of the ways you know, without looking, whether you are standing up or lying down. It also helps in balance while walking, and it is

what allows you to ride a bicycle. Even before your baby begins to walk, you can determine that vestibular function is intact by observing a reflex associated with this function.

How to Test Vestibular Function of the Inner Ear

1. Hold your baby in your arms at a thirty-degree angle (see the illustration).

2. Turn yourself in a complete circle in each direction. As you do, watch your baby's eyes. They should oscillate back and forth.

Any involuntary eye movement is called a nystagmus. The vestibular nystagmus, elicited in this way, indicates that your baby's vestibular function, or position sense, is in working order.

Children at Risk for Hearing Problems

It is possible to test hearing virtually from birth on and, surprisingly, an infant's hearing is every bit as keen as an adult's. But some infants are at greater risk than others of suffering from hearing problems. Five circumstances in particular pose increased risks to a newborn's hearing. If your baby falls into any of the following categories, you should be particularly alert for signs of a hearing deficiency.

1. *A family history of hereditary hearing disorders.* The key word here is *hereditary*—that is, a genetically determined hearing problem passed down from one generation to the next. A hearing loss in a parent or grandparent that resulted from injury or illness presents no risk to the next generation.

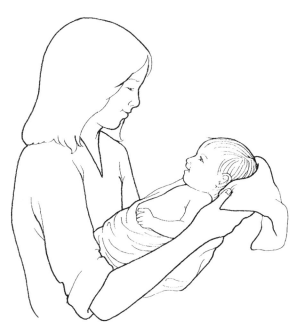

Testing vestibular function of the inner ear

2. *A history of German measles or other viral infection during the first three months of pregnancy.* Ordinary colds and sore throats don't count, and it is the first trimester of pregnancy that is the critical period.

3. *Defects or malformations of the ear, nose, throat, cleft lip, or cleft palate.*

4. *A birth weight of less than 1500 grams (3 pounds, 5 ounces).*

5. *Severe yellow jaundice within the first day or two of life.* A touch of jaundice developing in the first week of life is normal. Severe jaundice, however, that appears within the first day or two of life and imparts an orange hue to the skin is the culprit here.

Different techniques are used to test hearing at different ages. The younger the baby the more you will have to rely on your own judgment as to whether or not the baby has heard a particular sound. You will not be able to measure how sharply your baby hears; you can, however, satisfy yourself that your baby's hearing is intact or determine if a professional evaluation is in order.

How to Test Hearing in Infants

Two people are needed for this test—one to make test sounds and another to observe the baby's responses. Choose a time when your baby is wide awake and in a good humor. A sleepy baby or colicky baby will be less attentive and may not perform at his best.

1. In a quiet room, hold the baby on your lap facing you so that you have a good view of her face. Your partner should be positioned just behind the baby, taking care to be outside the baby's field of vision.

2. When the baby is preoccupied with your face or with a silent toy, such as a small stuffed animal, the unseen partner should make the test sound. Anything that produces a sharp not-too-loud noise will do fine—a squeaky toy, small bells, or rattles work well. The sound should be made to the right of the baby, then to the left; for infants six months or older, the sound should also be made from above and from below.

3. As the test sounds are made, the partner holding the baby should observe the baby's reactions closely. Depending on the baby's age, a positive response would be indicated by the following reactions:

Newborns: blinks eyes; breathes a bit faster; face brightens with increased attentiveness

Age three months: eyes widen; head turns slightly in the direction of the sound; baby exhibits a quieting, listening attitude

Age six months: turns head forty-five degrees or more in the direction of the sound and can usually tell whether the sound is coming from above or below

It is important not to produce false normal results by using test sounds that are too loud, such as blowing a whistle or banging on a pot within four to six feet of the baby. Many infants with significant hearing deficits do have some remaining hearing and will respond to very loud noises.

How to Test Hearing in Older Children

To take this test, a child should be at least three and able to respond well to your questions.

1. Use a small sound, such as a ticking watch, a CD player turned down until it's just barely audible up close, or tap the bottom of a paper cup with a cotton-tipped swab. See how far away the sound can be heard by a person known to have good hearing.

2. To test the child, start making the sound at a distance where you are sure the sound can't be heard. Have the child come gradually closer to the sound until he can just hear it.

3. Compare this distance with the distance at which the normal-hearing adult can hear the same sound.

Several things might lead you to suspect your child is unable to hear properly as early as six months, even outside of test situations. Babies do startle at sudden sounds and, later on, turn their heads toward sounds. A sleeping baby occasionally wakes to noises in the house. If this never happens, you should wonder why not.

Delayed speech development is another indication of a hearing problem. Tragic mistakes are made when a child who fails to talk is wrongly judged to be mentally retarded or autistic when the real problem is deafness. Seek professional audiologic testing for any child who fails to achieve the following milestones in speech development:

Three months: babbles and burbles

Four months: chuckles socially; makes guttural ah and oo sounds

Seven months: starts to say ma and da

Ten to fifteen months: says ma-ma and da-da and at least one other word

Fifteen to eighteen months: has a vocabulary of six to ten words that have meanings; begins putting together two- and three-word phrases

Two years: has a 100-word vocabulary and begins to use short sentences

Three years: talks in short sentences; uses plurals; may sing simple songs

Examining the Ears Using an Otoscope

The only part of the ear available for direct inspection is the external or outer ear—the shell of the ear, the ear lobe, the external ear canal leading into the head, and the eardrum at the end of it. In order to inspect the ear canal and the eardrum you will need an instrument called an otoscope.

An otoscope is a handheld instrument that enables an examiner to peer into the external ear canal or into the nose. This can be a valuable aid in identifying abnormal conditions that require medical attention, and it should be made part of your medical equipment. The device consists of a little funnel that is placed in the ear (or nose), a light arranged in such a way that it shines down the center of the funnel, and a magnifying lens. A professional-level otoscope can be purchased from medical supply stores starting at about fifty dollars, and less sophisticated models for home use are available in drugstores for about ten dollars. Considering how common ear problems are, it is a worthwhile investment. Some scopes are offered with an ophthalmoscope head for examining the eyes, but you don't need this. An ophthalmoscope is too difficult to use without extensive special training.

Ask your doctor or other health professional to show you how to use an otoscope, and do your first exam under his or her supervision. Practice on an adult first.

Some doctors recoil at the idea of a lay person using this simple flashlight device, and if this is the case with your doctor, our suggestion is that you don't insist and omit this test from your repertoire. The following instructions on how to use an otoscope are to be used only as a reminder after you have had your instruction and have practiced under professional supervision.

How to Use an Otoscope

1. The funnel that is attached to the otoscope head should be the largest size that will fit comfortably into the ear canal. If the funnel is too small, it will be very difficult to see anything; but for infants, the smaller sizes are appropriate.

2. The baby should be lying down with the side of the head resting comfortably against a pillow. Have an assistant gently restrain the baby.

3. Take hold of the shell of the ear about halfway down and pull it firmly backward. This straightens out the ear canal, which is normally bent just a little.

4. Switch on the otoscope light. Hold the instrument at its neck with the handle angling upward. Brace the hand holding the otoscope by placing your little finger on the child's head, using it as a prop. This way, any movement the child might make will push your hand and the otoscope away from the head.

5. *Before* you insert the otoscope tip, look into the ear to make sure there is nothing in the way. A careful examiner never pokes any kind of instrument into a body opening without watching where it is going. If at any point you encounter hard wax or a foreign object, stop the

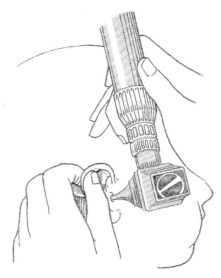

Using an otoscope

examination. The obstruction must be removed before proceeding further, and in the case of lodged foreign objects, this should be done by a professional.

6. Now, with the otoscope light switched on, insert the tip of the funnel just inside the ear canal. Under direct observation and still pulling backward on the shell of the ear, slowly insert the funnel down the ear canal until you can see the eardrum. Bear in mind that the total length of the ear canal in a baby or small child is less than half an inch.

What You Will See in a Healthy Eardrum

The eardrum is a slightly cone-shaped membrane stretched across the inner end of the ear canal. The eardrum gives the appearance of having a tent pole under it that makes a slight bulge in the center. A common error in ear examinations is to mistake the wall of the ear canal for the drum. Both are normally a light tan color with just a blush of pink. The eardrum, however, is a bit shiny compared to the canal wall and should reflect light back to you.

In order to recognize the subtle changes that indicate an ear infection, you must first be familiar with how the eardrum looks when your child is healthy. For this reason you should not wait until your child has an earache to inspect the canal for the first time.

But remember: don't proceed with an otoscope examination if there is hardened wax or a foreign object in the way. How you can recognize ear wax is described in the following section.

Recognizing Ear Problems and Infections

Ear problems of one kind or another occur frequently in childhood. You can learn to identify the most common of these complaints and sometimes deal with them yourself.

Ear Wax

As you conduct your otoscope examination you may observe ear wax in the canal. In an adult's ear, this is a dark, reddish brown material about the consistency and color of very thick automotive grease. In an infant's ears, ear wax is somewhat lighter in color. Sometimes the wax only partially obstructs the canal and you can complete your examination by looking past it. If, however, your view of the external auditory canal and the eardrum is entirely blocked by wax, you will have to have it removed by a health care professional. Once the doctor has cleaned and examined the ear, you may be given instructions on how to take care of wax problems yourself.

If a middle ear infection is suspected (see later in this section), you should not attempt to clean the ears of either wax or pus until a doctor has seen the baby and has provided instructions.

A Foreign Object or Live Insect in the Ear

Small foreign objects often find their way into a child's ear. Some objects such as small beads can be removed simply by turning the ear downward, gently pulling the shell of the ear backward to straighten the canal, and *gently* shaking the child's head. If you are lucky, the object will fall right out. If it doesn't come out easily, leave the removal to a doctor.

In the case of an insect, begin by killing it. Place two or three drops of rubbing alcohol into the ear canal. If rubbing alcohol is not immediately available, vodka or gin will do as well. Then the bug can be removed as any other foreign object. If the insect is visible without the aid of an otoscope, once it is killed it can be removed by grasping it with a small blunt-nosed tweezer. **However, never

insert the tweezers into the ear further than you can see the location of the tips.**

Earache

An older child is able to tell you if one of her ears hurts, but recognizing earaches in babies and very young children requires a fair amount of perception on the parent's part.

One unmistakable symptom is pain. Earaches hurt, and your baby will scream alarmingly. Babies scream for other reasons besides earaches, of course, so you will have to look for additional signs that point to an ear problem. Has your baby been sniffling, sneezing, running a fever, or displaying other cold symptoms? Middle ear infections often follow a common cold, and if your baby has been sick recently, the Eustachian tube between the throat and the middle ear may be stuffed up and causing pain.

Have you noticed your baby rubbing or tugging at an ear? This is another clue suggesting an earache. Does your child have a history of ear problems? Some ear infections will recur. Last month's earache may be back again. Some children may get two, three, or four ear infections a year for several winters in a row, and then never get another one again after that.

Middle Ear Infections

In medical terms, a middle ear infection is called acute otitis media. (*Oto-*, as you probably have guessed by now, is a prefix taken from Greek that means ear.) Pain and fever often accompany a middle ear infection, but not always. Doctors have found that pain and fever may be absent in about 25 percent of ear infections, although your baby may feel the effects in other ways.

The child may become irritable for no apparent reason, eat poorly, sleep fitfully, fret and whine, or even have an unexplained bout of diarrhea. Because ear infections are so common in children, doctors will always take a look in the ears when a child seems uncomfortable or unwell.

When there is a middle ear infection, the "tenting" appearance of the eardrum is gone, and it looks like a smooth, bulging membrane. The drum may be entirely red or there may be a pinkish red fringe around the edge. Other times the eardrum may look gray, dull, or wrinkled.

Any ear infection should be seen by a doctor. Conventional treatment is with antibiotics, and in cases of severe buildup of pressure, the doctor may decide to make a small opening in the eardrum to allow fluid and other by-products of infection to drain. This opening usually heals more quickly and easily than one that has resulted from spontaneous rupture.

Pus exuding from the ear may indicate that a rupture of the eardrum has already occurred. Pain will lessen or disappear when an eardrum ruptures because the severe pressure has been relieved. But you should still see a doctor to have the infection treated and to check for proper healing of the eardrum.

If you have to wait to see the doctor for some reason, inhaling steam may help a bit. Sitting in the bathroom with the shower running on hot is the easiest way to do this. Acetaminophen or ibuprofen in a correct child-size dosage can help with the pain and any fever there might be. Do not use aspirin.

Serous Otitis Media

Rather than being an infection, as is the case with *acute* otitis media, serous otitis media is usually an allergic phenomenon where the Eustachian tubes clog and fluid accumulates in the middle ear. It occurs mostly in older children, especially when there is a respiratory allergy such as hay fever or reactions to dust, animal dander, and other materials. It may also arise after repeated and frequent ear infections.

Serous otitis media generally doesn't hurt, so there isn't likely to be an earache to alert you to the condition, and there is no fever. Your child may complain of noises in her ears, however—buzzing, popping, crackling, or ringing. You may notice your child doesn't seem to hear well, and a hearing test as described earlier in the chapter will be indicated. In some cases of serous otitis, hearing difficulty persists for so long, unnoticed, that speech difficulties develop.

When you look at your child's ears with an otoscope, the eardrum will look dull and gray, thickened or wrinkled; and it will have lost its healthy shininess.

A child may have a single occurrence of serious otitis or repeated episodes. When recurrences are frequent, as many as three episodes in a six-month period, your doctor may want to take steps to try to correct the condition.

External Otitis (Swimmer's Ear)

Infection of the external ear canal is another common cause of earache in children. External otitis usually results from swimming in pools that are poorly chlorinated or have the wrong acid balance—hence its popular name, swimmer's ear. Moderate pain and mild fever are its main symptoms. The walls of the ear canal are an angry red rather than their usual pinkish tan.

You can often treat swimmer's ear at home. Soak a tuft of cotton in diluted vinegar (1 part vinegar to 4 parts water), and insert it loosely in the ear canal. Change it every two hours. If there is pain and fever, acetaminophen or ibuprofen in an appropriate child-size dose can help. Be sure, however, that the pain and fever is related to the *external* ear canal, and if the condition does not clear up within a day or two, you should see your doctor since antibiotic therapy may be necessary.

A drop or two of rubbing alcohol in the ears before swimming may prevent swimmer's ear altogether. Rubbing alcohol is also effective in removing water from the ears. The alcohol mixes with the water and the mixture evaporates more quickly than water alone.

Fungus Infected Ears

Swimming in polluted water can also cause an infection in the external ear canal. Its primary symptom is a severe itching, and closer inspection usually reveals gray or black particles (fungi) in the ear canal. Like swimmer's ear, this condition often responds to treatment with diluted vinegar. Severe cases, however, should be seen by a physician.

Bleeding from the Ear

Occasionally, a child will scratch the surface of the ear canal with a stick or other object. The skin of the ear canal is very thin, and even a small scratch may bleed profusely. Bleeding from the ear should never be ignored since it can be a sign of serious trouble after a head injury. For this reason, you should always investigate any bleeding from a child's ear to be sure it's coming from some small injury to the external ear.

If your child tells you he has scratched his ear, and otherwise seems all right, look into the ear with your otoscope. Remove any wet blood by twisting a tuft of cotton into a long cone and insert it into the ear to soak up the blood. **Do not use a cotton swab for this purpose; if something is in the ear canal, this will push it in further and may do serious damage.** Inspect the canal with your otoscope, watching as you go to be sure there are no foreign objects blocking the canal. If you find a scratch on the wall of the canal and the eardrum is intact, no treatment is necessary. These scratches heal by themselves.

Pierced Ears

It is unwise to pierce the ears of very young children because an earring may be grasped by another child in play and torn from the ear. This leaves a jagged laceration and the resulting scar may lead to a permanent ear lobe deformity.

If a baby or young child does have pierced ears, use only small stud earrings, a small ball or flat plate that fits flush against the ear lobe. Avoid loops or ornaments that project from the ear. Use only 14-karat solid gold posts (not plated or gold-filled); cheaper metals are apt to irritate the ears.

If the site of piercing becomes sore and tender, a minor infection has probably set in. It can usually be managed by keeping the retainer on the back of the post very loose, rotating the post at least four times a day and washing both sides of the ear lobe with alcohol. Application of antibacterial ointment after each cleaning can also be helpful. If the infection does not clear up within a few days, antibiotics may be necessary and the doctor should be consulted.

CHAPTER 6

HOW TO TEST YOUR BABY'S EYES AND VISION

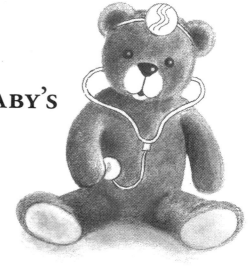

It is almost traditional to wait to check a child's vision until it's time to start school. Unfortunately, this is often too late. Some defects that can be corrected easily before age three are difficult and frequently impossible to correct by age five. So it is important for you to know something about how your baby's eyes work and how you can be sure his vision is developing the way it should.

How the Eyes Work

Both the eyes and ears can, in some ways, be thought of as extensions of the brain. And, indeed, these organs arise from the brain in a baby's earliest weeks of development in the womb.

The eye works much like a camera. At least the optical systems are comparable: both have a focusing lens system, an adjustable aperture for admitting light, and a light sensitive "film" at the back of a lightproof box. But that's where the comparison with a camera ends. In order to understand your child's visual process, you have to keep in mind that while a camera simply records pictures, eyes perceive—that is, the eyes and brain, working together, give meaning to the things we see.

While the perception part of vision is still largely a mystery, even to the experts, the optical or camera-like part is rather easy to understand. The body of the camera consists of the white of the eye, or sclera, the tough, fibrous tissue visible from the front and extending all the way around the eye to give it its global shape.

The lens system begins with the cornea. This is the clear, domed structure at the very front of the eye that you hardly notice when you look at the eye head on. If you look at the eye from the side, however, you can see how the cornea rises from the white of the eye at about the edge of the colored part and covers the front of the eye like a transparent cap. Light begins to be focused as it crosses the cornea, so any errors in its curvature, scars from an injury, or cloudiness from disease can have an important effect on vision. Injuries here are one of the most common causes of visual impairment in eye accidents.

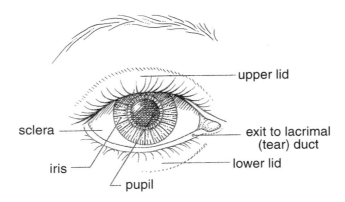

External structures of the eye

The colored part of the eye is the iris, which serves as the diaphragm for the optical mechanism, expanding and contracting to control the amount of light that enters the eye. The iris surrounds the pupil or entryway to the eye, which appears black because it is simply an opening in the iris, with the dark interior of the eyeball behind it. You can see the iris at work when light conditions suddenly become brighter, as when you go outside or when light shines in the eye. The iris diaphragm contracts, making the pupil smaller.

The main lens of the eye lies directly behind the iris. A ring of muscles around the lens contracts when you look at near objects, causing the lens to become a bit fatter, increasing its focusing power. With aging, the lens loses most of its elasticity and cannot change its focusing power, so corrective lenses are needed for near viewing in chores such as sewing and reading. Youngsters don't have this problem. They have great focusing power that enables them to literally bury their noses in books and see just fine, while their parents are approaching the point in life when it is difficult to read a newspaper at arm's length.

There is a clear liquid, the aqueous humor, between the cornea and the lens. This liquid is continually draining and being replenished in a way that maintains constant pressure within the eyeball. It is when this system goes awry that pressure builds and the condition known as glaucoma results. Glaucoma is unusual in children, though it can occur in babies born with an undeveloped eye-drainage system.

Behind the lens, the eye is filled with a clear jellylike substance called the vitreous humor. This, with the aqueous humor, maintains the global shape of the eye. The vitreous humor also provides part of the light-focusing power of the eye's optical system.

In order to see clearly, light must focus precisely on the retina, a light-sensitive membrane at the back of the eye. The retina is made up mostly of modified nerve cells that respond to light stimuli. These cells are called rods and cones. There is a small central area of the retina, called the macula, where rods and cones concentrate most densely. Sharpest vision occurs here, and the eyes shift constantly to keep as much light as possible focused on this area. There are many more rods than cones outside the macular area. The rods are most effective for seeing in reduced light, but they do not perceive color very well. That is why things appear in shades of gray at twilight, at night, or in a darkened room. And though you may not be aware of it, you cannot see colors of objects very well that are seen from the sides or corners of your eyes.

The most common problems of seeing—nearsightedness, farsightedness, and astigmatism—result from some fault in the eye's optical system. Images don't focus precisely on the retina, causing blurred vision or causing the muscles around the eye's lens to work harder than they should. These problems can nearly always be corrected with eyeglasses or other lenses, which help the eye's optical system to focus images more precisely.

Three pairs of muscles around each eye turn the eye up and down, from side to side, and diagonally. Under normal conditions, the eyes turn together to look in the same direction, giving binocular vision. But, as you will see, eye turning is not always well coordinated in babies and is one of the common problems you should be aware of and be able to identify.

Examining the Eyes

A baby's eyes are not completely developed at birth. Most babies are quite farsighted, the nerve cells of the retina are poorly developed, and the eyeball itself has a lot of growing to do before the power of the eye's lens and the size of the eye work together as an effective optical system. Even the pigment of the iris is undeveloped in the early months, which is why many white babies start out with blue eyes even though they may be destined to have brown eyes later. Coordination of eye muscles is not well established at birth, and many young babies (under four months) normally have occasional wandering or jerky movements of the eyes.

The most that you want to establish with a newborn is that sight is present and the eyes are

acting as they should at this point (see Chapter 1, "The First Examination of Your Newborn Baby").

How to Examine the Eyes of a Newborn

A small flashlight is all you will need.

1. Look at the eyes. The eyelids of a newborn are usually a bit swollen for the first day or two. Most of the time, a baby will keep his eyes shut tight.

2. Check the eyes when they are open. The eyes should be symmetrical (alike) in size, shape, and placement. The sclera (white part) should look white and clear, although babies with dark skin may have tiny black marks on the sclera, which are normal.

3. Check for vision. Shine your light at the baby's eyes, just momentarily, when she is awake and alert. A tight blink and an annoyed frown indicate the baby can perceive light. Some babies will try to follow a light that is directly in their line of vision, but don't expect this during the first week when vision and eye coordination are especially poor.

4. Check the cornea. Shine your light on the eye from the side. The corneal dome above the iris should be perfectly clear and transparent—with no spots, lines, or cloudiness.

5. Check the pupillary reflex. As described earlier, the iris constricts the eye's opening (the pupil) when light entering the eye increases. The pupil becomes smaller. When you shine your flashlight into the baby's eye briefly to check for vision and clarity of the cornea, also watch the

pupil. It should become smaller. Both pupils get smaller even though light is directed into only one eye. Check both eyes.

Eye Coordination

Eye muscle coordination develops within the first two months and should be well established by baby's fourth or fifth month. Eye muscles are coordinated when both eyes direct their gaze at the same place at the same time. This gives conjugate or binocular vision.

Strabismus

When only one eye looks at an object and the other eye wanders somewhere else, the condition is called strabismus; it should be brought to the attention of an eye specialist and treated as early as possible.

There are two kinds of eye specialists who treat this condition: an optometrist and an ophthalmologist. The optometrist has an O.D. degree (doctor of optometry) and cannot use medicines or surgery in treatments. The optometrist can treat strabismus with glasses, by covering one eye with a patch, or with exercises when a child is old enough to cooperate. An ophthalmologist is a physician with an M.D. degree (doctor of medicine) and a specialty in diagnosing and treating diseases of the eye. The ophthalmologist might use any of the treatments available to the optometrist, or she might opt for muscle surgery. There is often some disagreement between the two professions, although in many modern eye practices, ophthalmologists and optometrists work together.

If the eyes point even in slightly different directions, the child may see two different images. This is essentially what happens when a person's eyes dissociate and "see double" in a disease or drug-induced state (including an alcoholic state). Rather than be confused by two images, the brain tends to suppress vision in one eye. Vision in the unused eye soon begins to deteriorate. That's why it is important to see that strabismus is detected and treated promptly.

There is a most insidious old wives' tale that says an eye will straighten by itself and can be left alone at least until the child starts school. *This is not true!* If, at age four months, your baby has an eye that is turned continuously in or out (cross-eyed or wall-eyed), you should consult an eye specialist. If, at six months, one of your baby's eyes drifts away from the gaze of the other, consult an eye specialist. Don't let anyone tell you the child will outgrow it, and don't wait for treatment until the child is older. **Waiting can result in permanent loss of vision or impairment of the suppressed eye.** Trying to correct a muscle imbalance after age three is often impossible.

How to Test Eye Coordination

There are three ways to check for eye coordination. Try at least two of the tests.

1. Light Reflection Test. This is the easiest of the three tests to do, especially with young babies. Shine a small flashlight with a sharp beam toward the baby's eyes. The light reflection should be in the same place in both eyes. It will be centered in the pupils if the baby is looking directly at the light. If the light reflection is not in the same place in both eyes, the eyes are not gazing in the same direction; they are not aligned.

2. The Cover Test. Attract the baby's attention to a light or a brightly colored toy. Then cover

one eye with a card or your hand. As you cover the eye, watch the uncovered eye. It should not move as you cover the other eye. If it does move, it means that the baby was looking at the object with only one eye and he has to shift eyes when one is covered. Do the procedure again, this time covering the other eye. Try the test at two distances: first with the light or toy at about one foot, then at about two feet.

3. The Alternate Cover Test. Cover one eye with a card or your hand. Attract the baby's attention with a light or a brightly colored toy. While his gaze is fixed on the object, quickly uncover the eye. Watch the eye you have covered as you uncover it. It should not move. If it does move, it means the eyes are not working together.

A few children may develop an abnormal eye movement called nystagmus. This is a rhythmic, jerking eye movement. The eye usually moves quickly to one side and slowly returns. The eye may also move vertically or even in a circle. Nystagmus is common in newborns, but any remaining nystagmus after a few weeks or nystagmus that develops later should be reported to the doctor because it may be a symptom of a disorder of the nervous system.

Visual Acuity

Visual acuity refers to sharpness or keenness of vision. Like most other measures of human function or capacity, "normal" vision is measured against averages. If you meet the well-known standard of 20/20 for keen vision, it simply means that you can see objects at twenty feet as clearly as a lot of other people do.

If your vision is rated at 20/30, you have to be at twenty feet to see what a person with "normal" vision can see at thirty feet. But most people can get along very well with 20/30 or even 20/40 vision, depending on how they must use their eyes in their work and in leisure-time occupations. Something worse than 20/40 is likely to be uncomfortable and put you at a disadvantage in the everyday world.

Visual acuity is measured using any one of several standardized charts. The most familiar is the Snellen chart with the large E at the top and lines of letters that get progressively smaller as you move down. Other charts have been developed for very young children who don't know their A, B, Cs. We will talk about them at some length in a moment.

The undeveloped eye of a newborn sees rather poorly. All that you can expect to determine in an infant is that the eyes are in working order and perceiving light. After a few months, you can check for strabismus. When the baby is about two, you can begin to test for visual acuity. Visual acuity remains relatively poor for the first few years, reaching about 20/50 by age three, and 20/30 or 20/40 by age four. The adult norm of 20/20 isn't achieved by most children until some time between ages six and eight. Eye growth and development don't stabilize until age twelve or later.

Eye testing, however, should begin in baby's early months and should continue throughout life. It is important to know several things:

- Are the eyes working together?

- Is visual acuity about the same in both eyes?

- Is the child seeing as sharply as can be expected for his age?

- Is the field of vision as large as it is for others?

- Is there anything in the eyes that interferes with seeing?

- Is the child comfortable while seeing?

A child isn't aware of visual problems unless there is some pain associated with it, and there usually isn't. As far as a child is concerned, the way he sees the world is the way it is. If something is amiss, it's up to the parents to find out.

Testing Visual Acuity in Preschoolers

There are two kinds of charts for eye testing that can be used with children before they know numbers or the alphabet: the tumbling E test and the picture test. Eye-test charts can be obtained inexpensively from most medical supply stores or by contacting Prevent Blindness America at 500 East Remington Rd., Schaumburg, IL 60173; 800-331-2020. This organization will provide single tests for one child at home or instructions for a screening program that you may wish to establish in a community nursery school or other group.

The tumbling E test is easiest to do with older children, but you'll probably have to use a picture test for children under three. A precocious two-year-old is probably the youngest child you can test with any chart. The child must be able to communicate fairly well and cooperate in a "game."

Read through the instructions for the tumbling E test even if you don't use it. Some of these instructions apply to both tests. Be very patient with the child, making the test a game. If the child is cranky or reluctant, end on a cheerful note and try another time. Everything must be explained in advance and practiced before the test begins. One subterfuge that often works is to have two adults or older children play the game while the child to be tested watches. As the child becomes eager to play, too, bring him into the game.

Always begin by sitting down with the child as if you were telling a story. In a relaxed and friendly conversation, talk about the pictures or the "fingers" of the E and how they are used in the game.

How to Use the Tumbling E Test

1. Teach your child to point one or more fingers in the same direction the "fingers" of the E are pointing. Turn the E up, down, and to either side while the child points.

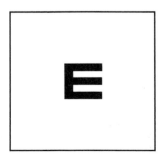

Tumbling E for eye testing

2. Cover one eye. You will want to prepare this part of the game in advance, too. There are several ways to do it. If the child is cooperative enough to hold a card or paper cup over one eye without peeking, this is a good way. A cloth or small stuffed toy held to one eye works as well, or you can try playing pirate and draping a Captain Kidd bandana over one of the child's eyes. However you do it, the rule is no peeking with the covered eye.

3. When your child has the idea, hold the E fifteen feet away in bright light.

4. Turn the E six times so its fingers point in different directions—up, down, and to the sides. Ask the child which way the fingers of the E are pointing. Have him show you by pointing his own fingers in the same direction.

5. If the child misses more than two of the positions, consider the test not passed. Move closer,

Picture chart for eye testing

two feet at a time, until the child can pass the test easily. Note the distance at which the test is passed with that eye.

6. Check the other eye and note the distance.

How to Use the Picture Test

1. Let your child see all the pictures at close range with both eyes. Be sure both of you understand the names of the pictures. The bear may be Winnie if the child has a toy by that name. The horse may be better known to him as a doggy, or a doggy a horse. Don't argue the point.

2. Cover one eye in any of the ways suggested for the tumbling E test.

3. Hold the pictures in good light at ten feet. Point to the pictures in random order and ask the child what they are. He should recognize them all easily. If not, move closer and try again.

4. Record the farthest distance the child can see the pictures easily.

5. Check the other eye and note the distance.

Evaluating the Results of the Visual Acuity Tests

Whatever the results of these tests, it is important that both eyes are performing about the same. If there is as much as a two-foot difference in the distance at which each eye passes the test, consult an eye specialist. If one eye is not seeing as well as the other, the brain tends to suppress vision in that eye. If steps are not taken to correct this, vision may be permanently impaired or lost in the suppressed eye. This condition is known as amblyopia, or "lazy eye."

Children of four and five should pass the tumbling E test at fifteen feet with both eyes; at age three to four, ten feet is okay. At three and under, eight feet is okay. If you get results at all with a two-year-old, simply determine that both eyes are seeing alike. If performance is not this good, or if the eyes are seeing differently, a professional examination is called for.

Peripheral Vision and Visual Field

Clearest vision is obtained when you look straight ahead at an object. That's because when you look at something straight on, light from the object falls on the macula, the most sensitive part of the retina. Perception of objects outside of a straight line of vision falls off sharply.

But from experience, you know you can be visually aware of objects far to the side of your direct line of sight. This is called your peripheral vision. It is not sharp vision; at the very edges, it is no more than perception of a shadow or a movement. Nevertheless, it is very important vision when you are driving, and in other potentially dangerous situations. How far to the side you can see, how large an angle up or down when you are looking straight ahead, is called your visual field. Loss of peripheral vision—a shrinking of the visual field—is a signal that something is wrong in the eye itself or in the nervous system that serves it.

How to Test Peripheral Vision

You can begin to test peripheral vision in your child at about age two, or as soon as the child will concentrate on things going on directly in front of her. Here is a simple test you can use with any child old enough to concentrate on a TV show.

1. Watch a favorite TV show with your child. Sit just in back of her on the floor or make her comfortable in your lap.

2. Have a hand puppet or small stuffed toy hidden but handy.

3. Wait until the child is watching the television with rapt attention—that is, staring straight ahead at the TV and rather oblivious of your presence.

4. Bring the toy from in back over the child's shoulder, wiggling it as you come closer. When the toy comes into the child's visual field, she will almost certainly turn to see what's going on, or she might slap at the toy with her hand. This should happen when you get just forward of the child's shoulder.

5. After some delay, when the child is not expecting the trick to be repeated, bring the toy down in front of the child from a point high overhead. She should catch sight of the toy when it's about level with the top of her head.

6. Try the test at intervals on both sides of the head. If you can manage to play pirate and drape a bandana over one of her eyes, you can test one eye at a time.

7. If the child doesn't notice the moving toy until it is well forward of the shoulder, or almost in front when you bring the toy down from above, check with your doctor. Try the test several times before you become concerned, however, and assess the general condition of your child's eyes, using the checklist at the end of this chapter.

Foreign Bodies in the Eye

One of the most common eye problems encountered by parents is a foreign body in the eye. Specks of dirt and sand are the most common offenders. Less common, fortunately, are flakes of broken glass, metal, and other hard objects that become lodged in some part of the eye as the result of an accident. Such foreign bodies, which adhere to the eye, or penetrate the eyeball or cornea, must receive prompt medical attention. Medical help should also be sought quickly if some chemical agent or caustic liquid has splashed into the eyes; but in this case, **immediate first aid—copious washing—must be administered before you even think about finding a doctor.**

How to Deal with Foreign Bodies in the Eye

1. Inspect the eye to see what you are dealing with.

   - Can you see the object?

   - Does the object seem loose and floating?

   - Is the object stuck or has it penetrated the eye?

   - Are there cuts, lines, or scratches on the eyeball? On the cornea?

   - Is there bleeding in or on the eye itself?

2. Review and evaluate the situation.

   - Where has the child been?

   - What has he been playing with?

- Could glass or sharp metal slivers be involved?

- Could dangerous liquids or solid chemicals be involved?

3. Use the appropriate procedure as described next in this section.

Familiarize yourself with the following procedures before you need them so that you can decide in relative calm whether you will deal with the foreign substance yourself or seek medical help.

Sand or Dirt

Wash the eye with plain, lukewarm tap water. You will probably need an assistant. Hold the eye open and wash with *gently* flowing water. Pour water *slowly and gently* from a cup or pitcher. One of the best ways is to squeeze water *gently* from a bulb syringe. With a syringe, you can direct the flow of water under the lids, which is most helpful in dislodging foreign bodies. If the child is old enough and will cooperate, have him put his head in a pan of water and blink.

Stuck, Sharp, or Penetrating Objects

Get medical help at once. Keep the child's hands away from the eyes. Restrain his hands if necessary. If the object does not seem stuck in the eye, try shaking it out. With the face pointed toward the ground, tell the child to give his head a good shake. Then wash and see a doctor to be sure no damage has been done.

Liquid or Solid Chemicals

Wash the eyes at once. Don't waste time going for help. Don't stop to find an eyewashing cup or syringe. Get to the nearest water and wash the eye. Flood it with water—gently, of course. For most chemicals, the eye should be washed a full five minutes by the clock. For acid splashed in the eye, wash ten minutes. Alkalis are even more dangerous than acid. Wash for twenty minutes. Lye, other drain cleaners, and some cement products contain caustic alkalis. Read labels and know what you have around. **After you have washed the eye, get medical advice.** Do not use vinegar, neutralizing agents, ointments, or eye drops—just water.

Evaluating a Blow to the Eye

Blows to the eye are frightening because of our natural fear of blindness. The sight of blood is also disturbing. But the eye is well couched in protective surroundings of bone, and the eyeball itself is very tough and resilient. Most blows in the vicinity of the eye injure the brow or cheek under the eye rather than the eye itself. At the same time, keep in mind that trauma (injury) is the most common cause of blindness in children over two. Take a moment to evaluate the situation. Cuts on the eyebrow or forehead can bleed mightily into the eye, giving the appearance that things are worse than they really are. Wipe away blood with a wet cloth to see where the blood is coming from and how bad the injury is. If it is a small cut or scrape on the eyebrow, treat it as you would other small injuries. But be alert for other symptoms of distress, as described in the following list.

You should get medical help

- if there is any injury to the eyeball itself—cuts on the white of the eye, scratches on the cornea. The cornea doesn't bleed, but injuries here are extremely serious nevertheless.

- if there is persistent pain or the feeling that something is in the eye, even if you can't find anything

- if there is bleeding inside the eyeball. This appears as severe discoloration in back of the cornea. It can often be seen in good room light or daylight, but check using a flashlight to be sure.

- if the eye has been struck by a small, fast-moving object, such as a pellet, BB, or stone

- if there is constant tearing or blinking long after the accident

- if the child continues to complain of pain, discomfort, blurring, or double vision, even though you can't see an obvious injury

- if an insect sting on the lid has swollen the eye shut

How to Treat a Black Eye

A black eye is caused by bleeding into the tissues around the eye, which causes swelling and discoloration. Using a flashlight, inspect the child's eye carefully. Be sure there is no sign of bleeding within the eye or other signs of injury as discussed above. If the only injury seems to be to tissue around the eye and if there is no bleeding from a cut or other wound, proceed as follows:

1. Apply ice to reduce swelling. Use an ice bag, or place several ice cubes in a plastic sandwich bag or freezer bag.

2. Have the child keep the ice in place for about a half hour at a time. Do this four or five

times in the twenty-four hours following the injury.

3. When the swelling has subsided, there will be some discoloration, which will disappear in time.

Conjunctivitis, or Pink Eye

The conjunctiva is the mucous membrane that lines the insides of the eyelids and extends to the white part of the eye. Under normal circumstances, the membrane that covers the eyelids is pink and glossy. Red eyelids and bloodshot eyes are very common in childhood and are most often caused by conjunctivitis, an inflammation of the conjunctiva. Its common name is pink eye.

Conjunctivitis is most frequently due to a minor viral infection, often part of a cold. It is not a serious condition and usually goes away when the cold does. But other things can cause eye redness, of course. It can occur with hay fever or other allergies, it can come from swimming in heavily chlorinated water or from an infection picked up in the water while swimming. It can also come from heavy industrial smog.

The usual pink eye is associated with a thin, watery discharge that may cause some yellow crusting first thing in the morning. A thick yellow or green discharge is a more serious matter, and if this occurs, you should take the child to see a doctor. You should also have medical attention if the eyelids become substantially swollen or if the redness lasts for as long as a week.

If there is constant tearing or blinking or if the eye has suffered a blow, consult a doctor. Pain or blurred vision with the redness should be called to a doctor's attention. And if the baby is less than a month old, you should make an appointment to see the doctor at once.

Children with simple red eyes, however, can be made more comfortable at home while the conjunctivitis is resolving itself.

How to Deal with Pink Eye

1. Wash the eyes frequently with warm (not hot) water—as often as every two or three hours while the child is awake. Squeeze the water into the eyes from a cotton ball as you hold the eyelids apart. Then sponge any caked material from the lids and lashes while the eye is closed.

2. Keep reminding your child not to rub his eyes. Some rubbing is expected and impossible to stop. Don't fret over it. Remind your child pleasantly that it's bad for his eyes.

A green or yellow discharge of pus from the eye indicates there is a bacterial infection and this should be seen by a doctor. The doctor will probably prescribe frequent cleaning and antibiotic eye drops. Ask your doctor to demonstrate a good way to administer eye drops if you haven't done it before.

How to Use Eye Drops

1. The child should be lying on her back. Gently restrain a small, uncooperative child. Explain what you are about to do, and reassure the child that the drops will just cause her to blink and be uncomfortable for a second or two.

2. Rest the hand that holds the eyedropper on the child's forehead. This assures accuracy of aim if the child is wiggling, and it keeps the dropper from hitting the eye accidentally.

3. Gently separate the eyelids with your thumb and forefinger.

4. Drop the prescribed amount of medication into the lower lid.

5. An alternate method is to pull the lower lid down and out to form a cup. Take the skin of the lower lid gently between your fingertips. Pull gently to form the cup and drop the medication into this.

How to Deal with Allergic Reactions That Affect the Eyes

Typically, the onset of an allergic reaction involving the eyes goes like this: Your child goes out to play on a nice spring day. Later, he comes in with his eyes reddened, irritated, tearing, and itchy. There may be some swelling of the eyelids. Ask a few questions to be sure he hasn't gotten some irritant in his eyes—sand, soapy water, or any of the other things kids find to get into. Eliminating other irritants, there could be an allergy at work, probably due to pollen in the air.

1. Wash the eyes with lukewarm to cool water. Hold the eye open and pour lots of water, gently, from a pitcher. This is best done with the child lying on his back. After washing, instruct the child not to touch his eyes until you have cleaned the rest of him.

2. Remove all clothing and wash it at once. Give the child a thorough shower and shampooing to get rid of all pollen that may be stuck to him or his hair.

3. If the eyes are still irritated, cool them with cold compresses. Use two clean washcloths and

a bowl of ice water. Wet the cloths and wring one out partially, leaving the other in the bowl. Place the cloth over both closed eyes. After about one minute, exchange cloths. Continue this for about fifteen minutes.

4. If the child is still uncomfortable, try one of the nonprescription eye drops that are recommended for clearing bloodshot eyes. Your pharmacist can recommend any one of several. Follow the directions on the label. You will find instructions for instilling eye drops in the preceding section.

5. Oral antihistamines also help relieve itchy, allergy-reddened eyes. Ask your pharmacist for a suggestion, but avoid antihistamine preparations that contain scopolamine, which should be listed on the label. This can make the child excessively drowsy and is unnecessary for dealing with allergy. Even some antihistamines without scopolamine cause drowsiness, so bike riding and other activities that require the child to be alert should be avoided.

6. Consult a doctor if

   • the reaction is so severe it keeps your child from sleeping or playing

   • the eyelids are swollen closed or almost closed

   • little bulbous sacs of clear fluid are developing on the white of the eye

   • the child continues to complain that it feels as if something is in the eye, and the feeling becomes more severe in spite of your treatments to relieve the eye irritation

Blocked Tear Ducts

Tear ducts (lacrimal ducts) drain tears from the eyes into the nose. There are two tiny drainage holes at the corner of each eye on the nose side. You can see these as little black dots on the margins of the upper and lower lids just before the corner of the eye, one hole on each lid. Tears drain through these holes and into a lacrimal sac alongside the nose and then into the nose. When more tear water is produced than the drainage system can handle, the eyes "tear up" and overflow. You may also feel like blowing your nose because of all the tears draining into it.

If the drainage system is blocked, the eyes are watery all the time. If this is the only symptom, you can try treating the blockage with massage as described in the following how-to procedure. But the drainage system may also become infected, resulting in red and swollen eyelids and a swelling below the eye next to the nose. If there are signs of infection or of a yellow or green discharge, leave it alone and see your doctor. Consult a doctor, too, if your child reaches three months and still has watery eyes.

If one or the other of your infant's eyes are continually watering and if there are no signs of infection, it is probably a simple problem of the tear ducts being blocked with mucus or a collection of cells. Repeated periods of massage may help.

How to Deal with Blocked Tear Ducts

1. Wash your hands thoroughly.

2. Inspect the eyes for signs of infection: pus, red and swollen lids, a swelling below the eye. If

you see these signs, do not do anything more, but take your baby to the doctor.

3. Place your index finger just below the corner of the eye against the nose. Massage gently downward and into the nose.

4. Repeat the procedure every two hours over two days. You may have to repeat the procedure from time to time until your child is two or three months old. If the condition continues much beyond this, consult your doctor about it.

5. If a mucuslike material collects in the corner of the eye as you massage, carefully wipe it away with a ball of cotton. If the material is yellow green and puslike, stop the procedure and see your doctor.

Sties

A sty is an infection of the hair follicle around the base of an eyelash. The sty is a small, red, swollen spot on the edge of the lid. It will usually come to a head like a pimple within three days or so. You can deal with most sties by using warm compresses.

How to Deal with Sties

1. Prepare a bowl of water that is as warm as you can just comfortably stand to keep your hand in.

2. Use two clean washcloths. Soak them in the bowl of water. Wring one out partially, fold it, and place it on the eye.

3. After about one minute, change cloths.

4. Continue the soaks for about fifteen minutes. Do this four times a day.

5. Apply an antibacterial eye ointment to the sty after the soaking. Ask your pharmacist for a recommendation, telling him what you want it for. The ointment doesn't help cure the sty, but it helps to keep the infection from spreading.

6. A sty that is treated with hot soaks will usually come to a head within three days or so. It then looks like an angry red pimple with a white head. Keep applying the hot soaks until the head ruptures.

7. Gently wipe away the liquid matter that comes out of the sty and then apply more antibacterial ointment.

8. Some sties form quite deep inside the eyelid and don't resolve themselves easily. If a sty is very painful, causes considerable swelling of the eyelid, or does not come to a head in four days, consult your doctor.

An Eye-Care Checklist

- Test visual acuity. Visual acuity should be very nearly the same for both eyes. Check once a year and throughout life.

- Check for strabismus. Test at six months, one year, and each year after that. Watch for frowning, head tilting, closing one eye to see.

- Test peripheral vision at age three and once a year after that.

- Check for blurred vision. The visual acuity test is best for this, but other indicators include frowning, excessive blinking, squinting, eye rubbing, holding the head in an awkward way, bumping into things unreasonably often, being unable to see pictures in a book unless very close.

- Observe the condition of the eyes: clear whites, pink and glossy lid linings, no redness or swellings, corneas clear, no cloudiness in the eyes, eyes not watery without cause, no eye shake or jumping, eyes move together, pupils equal in size and responsive to changes in light.

- Your child should not be unusually sensitive to light. (Don't count a first exposure to bright light, when we all squint and adjust.)

- Eye complaints should be noted and reported to a doctor: pain, itching, burning, blurring, excessive eye rubbing, headaches, waving the hand to wipe away spots in front of eyes, scowling or making faces when seeing.

CHAPTER 7

HOW TO EXAMINE YOUR BABY'S NOSE, THROAT, AND NECK

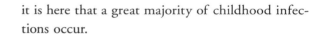

If you could peer far enough back into the nose, you would see a passageway descending to the back of the mouth. This is the pharynx, linking the mouth, nose, and throat. What we call the throat is, in fact, part of the pharynx. Air breathed in through the nose or mouth passes down the pharynx. Germs also travel up and down this conduit, which is why you almost invariably get both a sore throat and a runny nose when a common cold strikes.

The nose and mouth cavities are separated by the palate in the roof of the mouth, but become a common tube at the back of the throat. This shared passageway diverges into two tubes—the air tube (or trachea) and the food tube (esophagus). A flap of tissue, the epiglottis, protects the entrance to the trachea. When your baby swallows, the epiglottis seals off the trachea to keep food and liquids out of the air passageways.

The nose, mouth, throat, and trachea together are referred to as the upper respiratory tract, and it is here that a great majority of childhood infections occur.

How the Nose Works

The nose is the beginning of the upper respiratory tract. It delivers clean, humidified air to the lungs. As air swirls around the internal structures, it picks up moisture and passes through tiny hairs that screen out dust and impurities before being delivered to the lungs. Air is also taken in through the mouth, but it is more natural—and healthier—for your baby to breathe through his nose.

Obligate Nose Breathers

Some newborn infants, in fact, are obligate nose breathers—that is to say, they do not know yet how to breathe through their mouths. Even a mild cold or the sniffles can make breathing very difficult for these infants, so it is important to know if your baby falls into this category.

87

How to Tell if Your Baby Is an Obligate Nose Breather

1. To determine if your newborn is an obligate nose breather, simply pinch her nose closed for a few seconds (no longer!).

2. Observe whether she opens her mouth to take the next breath. If she struggles, fights, and fails to open her mouth, she's an obligate nose breather. If she cries, opens her mouth, takes a deep breath, and yells, she has already learned about mouth breathing.

If your infant is an obligate nose breather, keep the nasal openings clear at all times. In case of the sniffles, use a small rubber suction bulb, or aspirator, to remove nasal discharges. This will make her more comfortable, and within a few weeks the baby will learn to open her mouth when she wishes to take a deep breath.

Sense of Smell

Sensing odors is another important function of the nose. Sense of smell is controlled by the olfactory nerve. This nerve is actually a bundle of fibers that comes down directly through the base of the skull and into the roof of the nose. Odors reach the endings of these nerves from air coming in from the outside and from food vapors inside the mouth. This accounts, in part, for the loss of appetite that sometimes accompanies a cold. The stuffed-up nose cannot sense the odors of food as it is being chewed. Consequently food is less appetizing and eating less enjoyable.

The Sinuses

The nasal chamber also includes the sinus cavities. These are hollow pockets in the surrounding bone that connect with the nasal cavity via narrow passageways. There are three pairs of sinuses, but only one pair is significantly developed at birth. Since the sinuses are enclosed by bone, you will not be able to observe them in your examination of the nose. You can, however, appraise the external structure of your baby's nose and examine some of its internal structures by using a penlight.

Examining the Outside of the Nose

The basic shape of your nose is formed by a combination of bone and cartilage. Before examining your baby's nose, feel your own. Starting at your forehead, gently move your finger downward, pressing inward as you go. You will find solid bone as you pass over the bridge of the nose and down the ridge. As you proceed down, the bone gradually becomes softer until you reach the tip, where there is no bone at all but simply soft, flexible tissue.

A baby's nose has very little bone in comparison with an adult's. Because the center ridge of the nose descends from the forehead, it very quickly becomes soft and flexible. The bridge of the nose, moreover, tends to be somewhat flatter in black and Oriental babies.

Appraise the shape and position of your baby's nose. It should follow an imaginary vertical line drawn from between the eyes down to the center notch of the upper lip. The structure of the nose should be symmetrical, and the nostrils should be of equal size.

Examining the Inside of the Nose

You can examine the internal structure of your child's nose, using a flashlight or penlight. If you have purchased an otoscope for ear examinations (see Chapter 5), you probably have a nasal speculum, the largest of the little funnels that come with the otoscope. Somewhat shorter and fatter than the others, it is specially designed for looking into the nose. The combination funnel, magnifier, and light that makes up an otoscope lets you see a bit further into the nose. But it is not strictly necessary here.

When you look inside your baby's nose, you will observe three important features: the pink, spongy lining known as the nasal mucosa, the septum (dividing wall) and, a bit farther back, perhaps one of the conchae, or nasal turbinates. The conchae are three little chips of bone that protrude, shelflike, from the upper septum in each nostril. They are lined with nasal mucosa also and help warm and humidify cold, dry air.

How to Examine Your Baby's Internal Nose Structures

What you will be looking for are the color of the nasal mucosa, an intact septum, and any abnormal conditions such as swelling or discharges.

1. With the child's head tilted slightly back, push the tip of the nose upward and shine your light up into one of the nostrils. If you are using a nasal speculum, never insert the otoscope tip up the nostril without watching where you are going. Check to make sure that there are no foreign objects that could be pushed further into the nasal cavity by your speculum.

2. Inspect the nasal mucosa that lines the inside of the nose. This is normally pinkish, with a number of fine hairs.

3. Examine the central nasal septum, the wall between the two nostrils. The septum should be straight and smooth and divide the nostrils evenly. There should be no perforation of the septum. Check by shining your light into one nostril and see if light is admitted into the other. Light should not pass through the septum.

4. Look for the conchae. You may or may not be able to spot one of the three shelflike protrusions deep in each nostril. If you can, the nasal mucosa with which they are covered should be the same color as in the lower nostril.

5. Check for abnormal conditions. Normally, the nasal mucosa is covered with a thin, clear layer of mucus. When your child gets a cold or respiratory infection, this clear mucus turns yellow in a day or two and is secreted in great abundance. The nasal mucosa itself becomes reddened and swollen. During an allergic nasal reaction, however, the swollen membrane is pale, and the discharge, though profuse, is quite watery. Being out in the cold also stimulates a clear watery discharge as you know from your own experience of being outdoors in winter.

6. Repeat your examination with the other nostril.

Do your first nose examination when your baby is well. This will give you a basis for comparison when you fear that he is becoming ill.

Common Nose Problems

Nosebleeds

Nosebleeds are very common in childhood. They are usually caused by a combination of drying of the nasal mucosa and the normal sort of nose rubbing and picking that all children do. A blow to the nose may also trigger a nosebleed.

How to Deal with Nosebleeds

A nosebleed typically starts suddenly, with a dramatic gush of blood. The immediate treatment consists of stopping it with pressure. While you do this, the child should be sitting up and leaning slightly forward, to avoid breathing in blood that may be trickling down the throat.

1. Pinch the entire nose firmly between your thumb and forefinger. Instruct the child to breathe through the mouth. Put pressure on as large a part of the nose as possible. If you merely close up the nasal opening in the front, blood may back up into the throat without hindering the flow.

2. Exert moderate pressure for at least ten minutes by the clock. During this ten-minute period, do not release your pressure even for a moment to see if the bleeding has stopped. Firm clot formation takes some time, and you will simply disrupt this process and set yourself back by releasing the pressure before a full ten minutes has elapsed.

3. Give your child a small basin to spit blood into that may have run into the back of the throat. If bleeding has not stopped after ten minutes of pressure, try another ten-minute period. If a clot still has not formed, call your doctor immediately.

If your child has recurrent nosebleeds, tell the doctor. Sometimes it is helpful to rub a small amount of petroleum jelly inside each nostril once or twice daily to keep the mucosa soft. It may also be helpful to increase the humidity in the air in a child's room by putting a humidifier in the room at night. Avoid giving aspirin since aspirin affects blood clotting and can make it more difficult to stop a nosebleed.

Foreign Objects in the Nose

The nose is a favorite site for children to insert a foreign object—marbles, small plastic objects, peanuts, and hard peas, to name just a few. Unless an object is quite soft, it is generally unwise for you to attempt to remove it yourself. Soft objects, though, can be grabbed with round, blunt-nosed tweezers (not squared or pointed) and pulled out. Hard objects such as marbles are often very difficult to remove, and any attempt at retrieving them at home may only push them further in. If your baby forces a hard object up his nose, take him to the doctor.

Infected Hair Follicles

Some children develop infections of a hair follicle in the lower or front part of the nose. Nose picking can cause this, and so can plucking out nose hairs. A child with such an infection will have an exquisitely tender, firm, red lump, usually located just inside the nose.

Such small nose boils, whether internal or external, should never be punctured, squeezed, or pressed at home. They should always be seen by a physician. The blood in this area drains up toward the brain, and serious brain infections can result from improper management of these apparently minor infections.

Examining the Throat

Parents should have at least a passing familiarity with how their baby's mouth and throat look when he is well. Sore throats are common, and tonsils can become swollen. These and other problems can be identified and dealt with much sooner if you can recognize an abnormal condition when you see it.

You would think that examining a baby's throat would be a simple matter. No special tools are needed—a spoon or wooden tongue blade and a flashlight, at most—and it is, after all, simply a matter of looking in the mouth. However, you will find that it is not as easy as it seems. Babies and toddlers find it upsetting for anyone to be poking around in there. They won't stick their tongues out on command, neither will they say "ah-h-h" for you.

Pediatricians and nurses become adept at assessing the condition of the tonsils and throat with a very quick glance into the mouth of a screaming baby. You can catch a glimpse, too, whenever the opportunity presents itself. Other times you have to make the opportunity. Pinching the nostrils closed will compel a baby to open his mouth in order to breathe. (Don't try this, of course, with an obligate nose breather; see Obligate Nose Breathers, previously discussed in this chapter.) This affords you at least a limited view of the mouth and gives you the space to insert a tongue blade.

Using a Tongue Blade

A cooperative older child may not mind the tongue blade for just a moment or two. And if you use it to depress the side of the tongue instead of the center-back part, you will avoid eliciting the gag reflex and will minimize her discomfort.

On the other hand, the child may clamp her jaws closed and purse her lips around the blade. Trying to force the jaw downward using the tongue depressor as a lever won't work, and you may cause

a minor injury if the depressor splinters. Instead, hold the nostrils closed until she opens her mouth for a breath. At this point, advance the tongue blade in a bit further so that it touches the rear part of the tongue. This will stimulate the gag reflex and you will have a golden moment to make your inspection. Be sure your flashlight is on and ready.

If you have an assistant to help you, there's an easy way to immobilize a toddler for such an examination. With the baby lying on the bed, have your assistant bring the baby's arms up over her head. Hold the arms just below the elbows and pressed tightly against the sides of the head. This will prevent the baby from flipping her head from side to side.

All of this, as you might imagine, can be very traumatic for everyone, so you should have very good reason even to be looking at all. Better to acquaint yourself with your baby's mouth and throat as the opportunity presents itself, and save the guerilla tactics for when you suspect illness.

When a child is quite ill with a sore throat, and has a bad cough and difficulty breathing, the swollen structures of a sore throat can inhibit, even totally prevent, breathing. Therefore, **do not try to examine your child's throat if she is having any difficulty at all breathing.** Your efforts may set off a spasm that will make matters substantially worse.

The illustration describes what you'll see when you do get the chance to examine your baby's throat. Review this diagram first so your view inside the mouth will be an educated one.

How to Examine Your Baby's Throat

Using one of the stratagems as previously described to view the throat, you should be able to observe the following:

1. The inside of the mouth and the throat is lined with mucous membrane. This is normally wet and pinkish red in appearance.

2. Projecting down from the midline of the soft palate is a little flap of tissue—the uvula. When your baby swallows, the uvula acts as a flap, moving upward to close off the passageway to the nose. Once in a while, the uvula may have a small division in the center so that it looks almost as if two uvulas are present. This can be an entirely normal finding. But it can also be associated with a very small bony defect in the roof of the mouth. If you notice that your baby has this so-called double uvula, examine the hard palate by feeling the roof of his mouth with your finger. If there is a bony defect, you should be able to feel a soft, midline ridge in the roof of the mouth, which should be brought to your doctor's attention.

3. On either side of the uvula, there are little curved, almost curtainlike structures. These are the tonsillar pillars. Behind them, on either side, are the tonsils. In some children, the tonsils are small, and the edges barely protrude beyond the pillars. In others, particularly those who have had repeated throat infections, the tonsils become quite large and extend well into the throat cavity.

4. Behind the uvula is the back wall of the throat—the pharynx. It should be the same pink color as the tonsillar pillars. In a child with a cold, you may see a yellow substance running down this wall. This is mucus that has been secreted in the nose and is running down into the throat. Its only significance lies in the fact that the child has a bad cold.

It's helpful to practice examinations on a cooperative older child or an adult first so that you can learn to recognize the various structures. Then examine your baby's throat when he is well. The color of the mucous membranes is heightened during some illnesses, and it is important that you be able to judge when a color change has occurred.

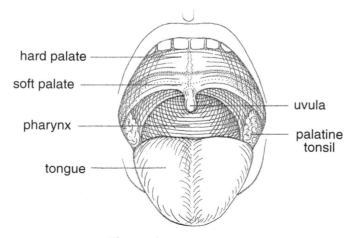

The mouth and upper throat

The Common Cold and Nasal Stuffiness

It is probably the most frequent infectious disease in any age group, and its incidence is even higher in early childhood. Common colds in children usually occur in epidemics that peak in early fall, after the opening of school, and in midwinter. Because they can be caused by many different viruses, colds vary in severity. The baby usually has a sudden onset of clear mucus running from the nose, a mild sore throat, a moderate fever, and sometimes a cough.

Many newborn babies have stuffy noses with mucus or clear discharges that bubble during feedings. The cause of this is unknown. It is probably not due to a viral disease and is not a cold the baby has caught during the first few days of life. The condition usually lasts two or three weeks and clears spontaneously.

A few babies under six months will have considerable difficulty breathing because of a cold. This is because they are obligate nose breathers (explained earlier in this chapter) who have not yet learned to breathe with the mouth open. **These babies and any baby under three months with a temperature of 100°F or more should be seen by a doctor the same day you find the fever.**

Most other common colds, however, can be managed at home. Try to relieve the symptoms that make your baby so miserable and be alert for signs that the infection is spreading rather than clearing up.

Fever

At the first sign of a cold, take your baby's temperature using one of the methods described in Chapter 13. The fever of a common cold is usually relatively low, rarely going higher than 102°F, but you should take measures to bring it down.

A tepid "towel bath" given right in the crib is a safe, effective method for reducing fever in a baby. Spread a large, absorbent towel over the mattress and place your baby, undressed, on top. Soak several washcloths in lukewarm water (about 80°F), wring them out, and bring them over to the crib. Place one of the washcloths on your baby's forehead, another under his back to lie on, and drape the other around the arms and legs and over his chest. Be sure to place a moist cloth between body surfaces that touch, such as between the thighs or between the arms and the chest.

Change the cloths as they begin to warm, and continue the "bath" for half an hour or so. At no point, however, allow your baby to become chilled. If he shivers or gets goose bumps, stop the treatment, as shivering simply generates additional body heat.

Afterward, gently rub your baby with a dry towel, dress him lightly, and recheck his temperature in a half hour. Offer cool liquids and reduce the room temperature, if possible. Extra fluids help avoid dehydration.

You may need to supplement these traditional measures with a fever-reducing drug such as acetaminophen or ibuprofen given in appropriate child-size dosage as indicated on the package labeling. But check with your doctor before giving fever-reducing medication to a child under two. Doctors advise parents to avoid giving aspirin to children with respiratory illnesses because of a suspected link between aspirin and the development of a rare condition called Reye's syndrome.

Fever-reducing drugs are not harmless. They can accumulate in a child's body and result in poisoning if they are given in excess. Check your child's temperature before repeating the dosage. If the fever is down to normal, skip the dosage. Take the child's temperature again later, and if the fever is back up, resume the medication.

If the fever-reducing medication fails to reduce the fever despite repeated doses (three or four prescribed doses over twelve to sixteen hours), then your baby may have something other than a common cold, and you should take him to the doctor.

Nasal Stuffiness

An infant's nose is easily blocked by the swelling and discharges that accompany a cold. Although an adult may find a stuffy nose merely annoying, it seems threatening to an infant, who prefers to breathe through his nose. And obligate nose breathers, as we have pointed out, know of no other way to breathe. Moreover, a baby cannot nurse and breathe through the mouth at the same time. Feeding becomes a frustrating ordeal punctuated by fitful stops and starts. You can help clear the nose using the following methods.

How to Administer Nose Drops

Nose drops can provide welcome relief to a stuffy baby. For a very young baby, nose drops are followed by suctioning the mucus as described in the next section.

1. Babies should be given only plain saline drops. These are made by mixing a quarter of a teaspoon of table salt in four ounces of water. How you administer the drops is important. You must get the solution to the back of the nose. To do this, the head must be at such an angle that the drops will flow back into the upper part of the nose.

2. With an infant, hold your baby in what nurses call the "football hold." Position her face up, between your arm and the side of your body. The palm of your hand should be under her head, supporting it. Tilt her downward at a slight angle so that the drops will flow back into the upper part of the nose.

3. Using an eye dropper, carefully squeeze two or three drops of the saline solution into each nostril. Keep holding your baby in the same position for a minute or two to allow the nose drops a chance to work. Then, gently remove any softened mucus using an infant nasal aspirator or an ear syringe. Squeeze the bulb, insert the tip gently into the nostril, and unsqueeze. This procedure should be administered shortly before feeding so that your baby enjoys its benefits when she needs them most.

4. For older children, have your child lie on his back on the bed, with his head hanging over the side. Administer three or four saline drops in each nostril. Again, wait a minute or two for the solution to soften the dried mucus, and then have him blow his nose. This can be repeated several times until the nose is clear.

MOIST AIR. Moist air soothes inflamed tissues in a stuffy nose and helps relieve congestion as well. Turn on the hot water in the shower and sit with your baby in the steamy bathroom for ten or fifteen minutes.

NOSE BLOWING AND SNIFFLING. Probably the best treatment for a runny nose is blowing the nose for a few days, if your child is old enough. Contrary to popular belief, sniffling and swallowing the mucus is not harmful. In fact, it may actually be beneficial in that vigorous nose blowing can force an infection into the ears. So if your child insists on sniffling instead of blowing his nose, he may actually be protecting his ears. In any case, sniffling and swallowing the mucus is neither dangerous nor injurious.

When to See the Doctor About a Cold

Usually, the progress of a cold is uneventful and its symptoms respond well to home treatment. There are a number of other situations, however, in which a baby with a cold should see the doctor, including the following:

- When there is an earache associated with the cold. The child may be developing a middle ear infection (see Chapter 5).

- When the discharge from the nose changes from watery or light yellow to a very dark yellow or green, and the dark-colored discharge persists for more than twenty-four hours. This may indicate that the child has developed a bacterial infection in addition to the viral cold. However, the nasal discharge due to a cold normally becomes slightly darker after naps or sleeping and lightens up again with activity. The nasal discharge of a child with a bacterial infection darkens and remains dark for twenty-four hours or more.

- When the nasal discharge persists for more than seven days or for more than forty-eight hours in a baby under one month

- When there is a fever that persists for four days or more

- When the skin under the nostrils becomes extremely raw or cracked

- When the eyes become crusted or watery

Finally, avoid over-the-counter combination cold remedies, and never give antibiotics without the advice of a physician. Never give a child an antibiotic you happen to have around the house with the mistaken idea that if it's good for one ailment, it must be good for everything. Even acetaminophen should only be used if the child has a fever, sore throat, or muscle aches.

"He's Always Sick"

A common problem in pediatric office practice is the child who is brought in with the complaint, "She has one cold after another" or "She's always sick." Although the problem is frustrating, approximately two-thirds of these children are simply having recurrent colds. In the preschool period, an average child has eight colds per year. Some children will have as many as twelve colds a year. Since these occur primarily in the months from September to May, this means that during the cold weather season, the child may have colds more frequently than once a month. It's frustrating, but not necessarily alarming.

Allergy

Many children who seem "always sick" with a runny nose may have an allergy. They may have hay fever, also called allergic rhinitis. The term "hay fever," however, is misleading—there is actually no fever involved, and it's more often caused by something other than hay.

The most obvious symptom is a profuse nasal discharge of a clear, mucouslike substance. Associated symptoms are frequent sneezing, rubbing the nose, and red, watery eyes. On examining the nose, you can see that the nasal conchae are swollen and appear slightly lighter than their normal color.

Hay fever most frequently occurs during the pollen seasons of the spring and early summer months. During late April and May, the most common offending pollens are from trees. From May through mid-July, the pollens are usually grasses. A second pollen season occurs from late August to mid-October, when ragweed pollen is the prime offender.

Any child with hay fever should be under a doctor's care, but there are a number of things which can be done at home. Used at your doctor's direction, antihistamine medications often are helpful and are usually more effective if started early in the attack. Your doctor will probably want to start with a simple nonprescription antihistamine from the drugstore.

Most children will not need to take antihistamines regularly throughout the pollen season. Sometimes once a day is plenty, and occasionally children can be well managed receiving antihistamines only when the air pollen count becomes unusually high. The main side effect is drowsiness, though tolerance to this develops within a week or two. Your doctor will be the best judge of which antihistamines to use and how often. If an older child with hay fever is going to participate in an activity such as hiking in the woods, which is likely to provide a particularly high pollen exposure, it is best to give him some antihistamine beforehand even though he has no symptoms.

The most effective management of hay fever is, of course, avoidance of the pollen or other allergen—which is not always easy. Pollen exposure can be reduced by not taking your child on drives or walks in the country and by staying indoors when it is windy and the pollen count is particularly high. Be sure to close the windows facing the prevailing winds. If possible, install a room air conditioner in the child's bedroom. There are also electrostatic precipitators available to filter bedroom air.

Pollen is quite sticky and tends to collect on exposed body surfaces, especially the hair. During pollen season, shower and shampoo your child every night before she goes to bed, and urge her to avoid handling pets whose hair has also collected substantial amounts of pollen.

Nose drops and nose sprays usually do not help in hay fever because the nasal secretions are so heavy they wash the medicine out shortly after it has been instilled.

Pollens are not the only allergens that produce allergic rhinitis in children. Many children are allergic to animal danders, particularly cat danders, which are small flakes of animal skin like human dandruff. Such conditions are usually very easily managed by just keeping the child away from the offending allergen. If this is impossible, work out a reasonable allergy control program with your doctor.

Sore Throat and Other Infections of the Respiratory Tract

There are many different varieties of sore throat caused by an assortment of germs. The catch-all medical term for them is pharyngitis, which simply means an infection of the pharynx, or the throat.

Within this broad category are problems such as tonsillitis, strep throat, laryngitis, epiglottitis, and so on, all of which are more specific terms indicating which part of the respiratory apparatus or what kind of germ is principally involved.

Since symptoms are similar and overlap from one condition to another, any sore throat should be seen by a doctor, especially when symptoms become obviously distressing or severe. Meanwhile, children with a sore throat can be made more comfortable by having them gargle with warm saltwater, suck on hard candy, and eat soft foods.

Most cases of sore throat, especially when they accompany a common cold, are mild, cause a minimum of discomfort, and clear up within a few days. Not all sore throats are as benign as this, however, and parents should be alert to the possibility of a more serious infection.

Although you don't want to panic every time your child has a sore throat with a common cold, keep in mind that some of these conditions can be dangerous, even fatal. Caution is the rule. Be alert for rapidly worsening symptoms, especially distress or difficulty when breathing.

Clearly, assessing a sore throat can be tricky. Symptoms overlap, and conditions can worsen rapidly. As we have cautioned before, the swollen structures of a sore throat can inhibit and even totally prevent breathing. Therefore, do not try to examine your child's throat if he is having any difficulty at all breathing. Your efforts may set off a spasm that will make matters substantially worse.

Finally, it is worth noting that some of the illnesses described below follow on the heels of a common cold or other respiratory tract infection. Any time your baby is recovering from an illness of this kind, only to suffer a relapse, see the doctor. If your child is too young to describe the symptoms being experienced, a visit to the doctor is in order.

Common Causes of Sore Throat and Their Symptoms

SIMPLE SORE THROAT. A simple sore throat may accompany or precede a common cold with its symptoms of sneezing and a runny nose. The child will likely be irritable and, if old enough, will complain of the hurt. It lasts less than five days. Bed rest, acetaminophen in a dose appropriate for the age of your child, soft foods (ice cream, gelatin, soups, liquids, and puddings), and a warm saltwater gargle for older children will help.

STREP THROAT OR TONSILLITIS. Both the throat and the tonsils are involved. It will likely be accompanied by a fever higher than you would expect with a simple sore throat (to 104°F). The sore throat will be severe and the child may also have a headache. The onset of the sore throat is abrupt, and you will see white patches on the throat and tonsils when you look. Lymph nodes in the neck will be enlarged (see "How to Examine Your Baby's Neck" later in this chapter). Since strep throat can affect other organs if left untreated, antibiotic treatment is required and you should see the doctor promptly.

PERITONSILLAR ABSCESS. It affects the area of the throat around the tonsils. There is high fever, swelling—usually on one side of the uvula—and lymph nodes of the neck are swollen. The child may have a nasal twang to her voice and be unable to open her jaw. This is one of the serious complications of an untreated strep throat. **It is a medical emergency and should be seen by a doctor at once.**

LARYNGITIS. This can follow on the heels of a cold and manifests as hoarseness, cough, and a slight fever. If the laryngitis is mild, then bed rest, moisture, and fever reducers should be enough. If it persists and becomes severe, you should take your baby to the doctor.

CROUP. Various kinds of croup can affect the larynx, the epiglottis, the trachea, and the lungs. There is a metallic or barking cough, and noisy or labored breathing. It can come on suddenly following an upper respiratory tract infection or when the child has had some other form of illness. In acute epiglottitis, or bacterial croup, breathing is noisy and difficult and the child may have an anxious, frightened look. He may assume a "tripod" position—sitting upright, leaning forward with chin out and mouth open in an effort to breathe.

Since it may be difficult to differentiate among the various kinds of croup, the doctor should be seen at once with any one of them. **If breathing becomes difficult at any time, such as with epiglottitis, it is a medical emergency and you should call for an ambulance.**

Anatomy of the Neck

The neck is a muscular structure with the bones of the spinal column running up the back in the middle. In the front of the neck, the trachea (windpipe) can be seen as a slightly bulging tube running up the midline. The trachea is supported by a series of cartilaginous rings that keep it semirigid and wide open for the free flow of air in and out of the lungs. At the upper end of the trachea is the

Adam's apple (cricoid cartilage), and just above this is the larynx, or voice box.

How to Examine Your Baby's Neck

1. Place your thumb and index finger on either side of the trachea and gently feel for any lumps or masses. As you move up and down the trachea, you will feel the cartilaginous rings that support it. The trachea should always be located in the midline. Any deviation to either side is not normal and should be brought to the doctor's attention promptly.

2. Locate the muscle mass that runs the length of either side of the neck. The cervical lymph nodes are distributed along this longitudinal muscle mass on both sides of the neck. You usually can't feel these under normal circumstances.

3. Feel for swollen lymph nodes. Using the flats of your fingertips, gently press with a circular motion along the area where these lymph nodes are located. But do not press on both sides at the same time. Your baby's head should be tilted upward just a bit, but relaxed and not tensed. Swollen lymph nodes are relatively hard and have sometimes been described as the size of a BB shot. Make note of any swollen lymph nodes you find in your examination. They may be tender, causing the child to wince or cry. Note if this is the case. These will be discussed in greater detail later in this chapter.

4. Finally, check for range of motion. Your baby should be able to tilt his head back to look at the ceiling, downward so that the chin touches the chest, and from side to side until the ear almost touches the shoulder. A young baby won't

be able to demonstrate all these maneuvers, of course, until neck strength is achieved. Check any questionable findings with the doctor, especially if your baby has other signs of illness.

Evaluating Your Findings

SWOLLEN LYMPH NODES. Enlarged lymph nodes are a sure sign that your baby is fighting off an infection of some kind. The lymph nodes are little nodules of tissue that function as filters. When the body has been invaded by infection, the lymph nodes trap bacteria, viruses, and other debris traveling through the bloodstream. As a node accumulates more and more of this material, it enlarges and you can feel it quite easily.

The body has a large number of lymph nodes. Besides those in the neck, there are nodes in the armpits, behind and above the elbows, in the area of the groin, and in the hollow of each collarbone. Different lymph nodes drain different parts of the body. Knowing which nodes filter which areas can help you to identify the probable source of an infection.

You are most likely to find swollen lymph nodes under your child's jaw. These nodes commonly swell as a reaction to a toothache, sores in the mouth, a cold, or flu. Swollen nodes behind the ears suggest German measles, an ear infection, or an infected tick or insect bite on the head. Enlarged nodes in front of the ears point to some problem in the area of the face or eyes. Swollen lymph nodes due to a localized infection are relatively hard, warm to the touch, and tender. As noted earlier, they have sometimes been described as the size of a BB shot, though some become considerably larger, reaching the size of a pea or even a small bean.

Swollen lymph nodes in a child with a cold or other respiratory infection, or in a child with an ear infection—particularly if the swollen lymph nodes are on the same side as the ear infection—are rarely a cause for concern. The source of the infection, of course, must be treated, but the lymph nodes will take care of themselves.

Swollen lymph nodes in an otherwise apparently healthy child, however, especially one who has not been ill recently, could indicate the beginnings of a serious disorder. If you find swollen lymph nodes in an otherwise healthy child, point this out to your physician.

STIFF NECK. Occasionally, an older child may hold her head turned to one side, with one shoulder slightly elevated. If this finding accompanies a respiratory infection such as a cold or flu, it is probably a simple stiff neck. One of the neck muscles is in spasm, pulling the head down to the side by its constant state of contraction. Treatment consists of acetaminophen for pain relief, and a heating pad or hot, moist towels to relax the muscles. The problem usually disappears in a day or two.

Stiff necks are rare in children younger than five, however. Moreover, a similar picture can occur following a neck injury. Because of the possibility of injury to the spinal column in the neck, children with suspected neck injuries should always be brought to the doctor promptly.

An infant or child who appears to be generally ill and who is unable to touch his chin to his chest is in need of immediate medical attention. The inability to touch the chin to the chest is one of the signs of meningitis, an infection of the covering of the brain or spinal cord. An apparently ill child with this finding should be treated as a medical emergency.

About Tonsillitis and Tonsillectomies

A large percentage of throat infections affect the tonsils. It's worth remembering, however, that the tonsils and the adenoids (which are actually another pair of tonsils located further up in the nasopharynx) are masses of lymphoid tissue with an important function. They help protect the trachea (air tube) and esophagus (food tube) from invading germs, and probably play a role in antibody formation as well. In other words, they are there for a reason. In fact, the body will attempt to regrow these tissues if they are removed.

This being the case, many of the reasons put forth in the past to justify their removal are being reexamined. Large tonsils are not bad tonsils, and enlargement of the tonsils even to relatively spectacular sizes is not in itself reason to remove them. Young children normally have larger tonsils than adolescents or adults, perhaps because they are more vulnerable to upper respiratory infections and have greater need of them.

Recurrent colds and sore throats also are not a reason to remove the tonsils. As noted earlier, some children will have respiratory infections as frequently as once a month or more, and removing the tonsils will not decrease the frequency or severity of viral respiratory infections. Neither will a tonsillectomy decrease the likelihood that your child will come down with strep throat. Although this was at one time thought to be a reason to remove tonsils, studies have shown that the incidence of streptococcal infections does not decrease after tonsils have been removed.

Completing the litany of excuses, poor appetite, unexplained fevers, bad breath, and noisy breathing are all equally poor reasons for removing the tonsils. If your doctor gives any of these reasons for recommending a tonsillectomy, he may be right, or he may have other reasons he hasn't mentioned. But it would be a good idea to get a second opinion before making a decision.

Now for the arguments in favor of tonsillectomy. The tonsils should be removed

- if they are so large there is actual obstruction, making it difficult for the child to swallow. This might be the case if the tonsils are so large they almost touch in the midline.

- if your child has recurrent peritonsillar abscesses

- if your child has recurrent bacterial infections in the lymph nodes of the neck or a suspected tumor of these nodes

The removal of adenoids, like the removal of tonsils, should also be done only under very specific conditions. Reasons for an adenoidectomy are persistent nose obstruction and mouth breathing. The child will also most likely have a nasal quality to her speech. To warrant adenoid removal, however, this must be a persistent and long-term problem. Continual nighttime snoring and daytime nasal snorting have been considered good enough reasons for adenoidectomy by some authorities. Finally, some authorities recommend the removal of adenoids in children with recurrent ear infections. However, most children with chronic ear infections do not have this condition due to large adenoids. Again, a second opinion is always a good idea.

CHAPTER 8

HOW TO EXAMINE YOUR BABY'S MOUTH AND TEETH

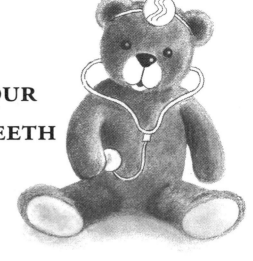

A baby explores the world with his mouth. The nourishing breast, the friendly pacifier, and the comforting thumb are among his first and most pleasurable experiences. Rattles, toys, and crib railings all find their way to your baby's mouth. And so—more or less—do a loaded spoon and a cup of juice. The mouth is one of your baby's most intimate connections with the world around him, and he makes the most of it.

Although examining your baby's throat can be a real challenge, the mouth is a bit more accessible. The tongue, the gums, and, later, the teeth can all be seen easily when your baby laughs, chortles, cries, and so on. For the other features of the mouth—the mucous membranes, the salivary ducts, the palate in the roof of the mouth—you may need your tongue blade and flashlight.

Review the guidelines in the previous chapter regarding the proper use of a tongue blade before beginning your inspection. Then try your examination. Don't feel you must cover all of the following features at one time. Check a few now, and save the rest for other inspections.

Examining the Tongue

The tongue dominates the scene in the mouth, but it should not protrude from the mouth. Normally it has a pink, rather rough look and is wet with saliva. It is the taste buds, or papillae, that give the tongue its rough texture. A coated or furry tongue is usually associated with mouth breathing, fever, or dehydration; it is also seen in children on soft or liquid diets.

An unusual, though by no means alarming, finding is smooth patches on the otherwise rough surface of the tongue. These patches can be circular or eliptical and are often surrounded by a narrow ring of slightly raised tissue. The condition is known as geographic tongue because of its vague resemblance to a contour map. This condition is rarely seen after age six. Geographic tongue is painless and, though it may last from months to years, it will eventually clear up by itself and requires no treatment.

Two other findings are deep, irregular grooves in the top surface of the tongue or a tongue that

101

seems too large and protrudes a bit from the mouth. Either of these may be perfectly normal in some children. Frequently, however, they are associated with Down's syndrome and indicate some degree of mental retardation. If you believe your child's tongue has either of these characateristics, bring it to the attention of your doctor.

There is a thin sheet of tissue underneath the tongue between the floor of the mouth and the middle of the underside of the tongue, called the frenulum. Its size and tightness vary greatly among children. It was once thought that a tight frenulum prevents the child from speaking and interferes with nursing, but this is rarely the case. A short frenulum in no way interferes with the ability to nurse, and it is unlikely that it will interfere with speech. If your baby can stick her tongue out and touch it to the roof of the mouth, the frenulum is just fine.

Examining the Cheek Walls and Gums

The side walls of the mouth cavity are lined with the same mucous membrane that lines the nose, throat, and other parts of the mouth. They are normally wet and pinkish red in appearance. If you look closely at either of the cheek walls inside the mouth, you can often see the point at which the salivary duct enters the mouth. This is a small, pimple-like opening at about the middle of the cheek wall, just below the level of the upper gum line. If salivary glands become infected, they appear red and swollen and the area is very tender. This condition should be brought to the attention of your doctor promptly.

An early sign of measles is small white flecks or spots scattered in the mucous membrane of the mouth, called Koplick spots. They are most easily seen by gently scraping the tongue blade across the surface of the mucous membrane and observing the area where the mucus has just been wiped away. Hopefully, few readers of this book will ever see Koplick spots because they will have had their children properly immunized against measles.

Next, look at your baby's gums. The mucous membrane covering the gums should have the stippled texture of orange peel. In dark-skinned babies, a brownish area defines the gum line from the rest of the mucous membrane.

If your baby is six months or older, chances are that teeth are already sprouting from the gum lines. A rule of thumb for babies two years and younger is "age in months minus six is equal to the number of teeth." More about teeth later.

Examining the Hard and Soft Palates

The arched roof of your baby's mouth consists of the hard palate near the front and the soft palate toward the back. It, too, is covered with mucous membrane and should appear dome shaped. Check the roof of the mouth with your finger. The hard palate should form an uninterrupted dome. If there is a midline ridge in the roof of the mouth, tell the doctor about your findings.

Common Mouth Problems

Drooling

At birth, the newborn does not secrete a great deal of saliva. At about age three months, however, the saliva flow begins to increase. Soon the flow of saliva outpaces the baby's poorly coordinated swallowing reflex, and the excess saliva drools out of the mouth. This is perfectly normal. Minor drooling that begins at age three or four months and continues for six or more months thereafter is not a cause for concern.

Teething, beginning around five months, aggravates the problem of drooling. So do painful sores in or around the mouth area. Drooling is not a sign of mental retardation. Although it is true that many mentally retarded children do a considerable amount of drooling, this is simply because it takes them longer to learn to swallow their saliva than it does normal children.

You should be concerned, however, if drooling seems to come on with a sore throat. It is possible that structures in the throat may be swollen, thus discouraging your baby from swallowing. If you have even the slightest suspicion that this may be the case, see a doctor at once.

Thrush

Bottle-fed babies sometimes develop a fungal infection of the mouth called thrush. This is caused by the same fungus that causes a candida (monilia) infection in a woman's vagina. Thrush consists of white, irregularly shaped patches on the mucous membranes inside the mouth, and, sometimes, the tongue. These flat, white lesions are often mistaken for milk but cannot be washed away. If you try to wipe lesions off with a wet washcloth, they're apt to start bleeding.

Thrush often occurs after mild abrasions of the inside of the mouth and is more common in children who have been receiving broad-spectrum antibiotics. It should be called to the doctor's attention so that treatment with an antifungal medicine (usually Nystatin) can begin.

Bad Breath

Continual bad breath in a child is not a disease in itself but, rather, an indication that something else is going on. A careful examination of the nose and mouth will often reveal the cause.

Acute infections of the mouth and throat can cause bad breath, as can acute infections of the nose. A more unusual cause of bad breath is a foreign body that a child has put in his nose, which has gone undetected for several days. Some children who are continual mouth breathers have bad breath; thumb sucking and blanket sucking occasionally lead to bad breath, too.

Good oral hygiene habits will generally clear up most cases of bad breath if the cause cannot be found by careful examination of the nose, mouth, and throat. If these measures do not take care of the problem, the child should be taken to the doctor or dentist for a more thorough evaluation.

Mouth Sores

Sores in the mouth fall into three categories: canker sores, herpes simplex, and cold sores.

A canker sore is a small, painful ulcer on the gums or on the inside surface of the lips. Canker sores usually occur only one or two at a time and are not associated with fever. They occur regularly in some children though their cause is not known. An allergic phenomenon is suspected, but this has not been proved.

Herpes simplex is a viral infection that produces lesions looking very much like canker sores. Children with herpes simplex develop multiple small ulcers of the mucous membranes. These may appear on the inside of the cheeks down to the tonsillar pillars of the throat and forward to the inner side of the lips. These ulcers may also appear on the tongue. Herpes simplex infections are usually associated with fever and with slightly enlarged and tender lymph nodes in the neck. There may also be a generalized reddening inside the mouth.

Canker sores are often mistaken for herpes simplex. The main difference is in the number of lesions and their location. Canker sores come singly or in pairs; herpes simplex produces multiple sores. Canker sores are usually limited to the inside of the lips, whereas herpes simplex spread farther back in the mouth.

For canker sores and mild herpes simplex infections, there are several things that can be done at home to make your child more comfortable. Massaging the mouth ulcers with a fruit-flavored brandy will deaden the pain a bit; this can be done three or four times daily. Acetaminophen will also relieve the pain somewhat. Modifying the diet may help. Allow your child to drink things like malted milk through a straw, and avoid offering salty or acid foods and things that need much chewing. Cold drinks, especially milk shakes, go down easily and provide considerable nourishment at the same time. With canker sores, try eliminating suspect foods, such as chocolate, nuts, and tomatoes. These are not proved offenders, but it's worth a try.

A child with severe herpes simplex should be seen by a physician because the discomfort will interfere with both eating and drinking. Dehydration may result if the child refuses to drink because of the painful mouth. So be sure to call your doctor if your child is not taking in adequate fluids. Also, call the doctor if the lesions last for more than one-and-a-half to two weeks or when the lesions are accompanied by fever or other symptoms. A prescription ointment is now available that can treat, though it doesn't cure, an initial herpes simplex infection.

Cold sores, also called fever blisters, occur on the outer portion of the lips. They generally last from one to two weeks and are also caused by the herpes virus. Applying alcohol to these blisters four times a day when they begin to dry will often speed the healing process. The alcohol will sting when being applied, however. Avoid softening ointments such as petroleum jelly. These hinder drying and healing. There are a number of over-the-counter treatments that can help. Ask your pharmacist for a recommendation.

Cold sores often occur in a susceptible child as a result of exposure to intense sunlight. If your child has a tendency to develop cold sores, apply one of the sunscreen lip balms with a high SPF (sun protection factor) number before sending him outside on a sunny day. Children with cold sores do tend to get them over and over again, however, and it is not possible to prevent all recurrences.

The Teeth

A most momentous finding is the first tooth that pokes up through the gumline in the front of the lower jaw. It is the first of the primary teeth, which are of primary importance.

Healthy primary teeth guide the permanent teeth into their proper positions. The untimely loss of a primary tooth due to injury or decay leaves an unnatural gap in the mouth. If other teeth are allowed to drift into these gaps, the permanent teeth will probably come in crooked. In the long run, the care you spend on your baby's primary teeth will be a worthwhile investment toward a healthy permanent set.

Whereas a full adult set of teeth numbers thirty-two, a baby will eventually have just twenty—ten in the upper jaw and ten in the lower.

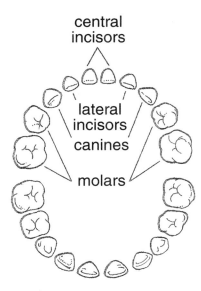

central
incisors

lateral
incisors

canines

molars

The primary teeth

Starting in front are the two central incisors; these are the first to erupt. The central incisors are flanked on either side by a lateral incisor and a canine. These are the next to show. Finally, the last teeth to appear are the two molars on either side in the back.

As the following chart shows, the first tooth breaks through at about six months, with teeth in the lower jaw generally appearing about six to eight weeks before their counterparts in the upper jaw.

This timetable can vary by as much as six months to a year and still be considered normal. Any greater deviation from this schedule, however, should be brought to the attention of a dentist.

Caring for Your Baby's Teeth

By the time all the primary teeth are in—roughly age two—your child should begin seeing a dentist regularly. Even before this, however, you should be

Average Ages of Eruption and Loss of Primary Teeth

Teeth	Lower Jaw	Upper Jaw	Age of Loss
Central incisors	6 months	7 months	7th year
Lateral incisors	7 months	9 months	8th year
First molars	12 months	14 months	10th year
Canines	16 months	18 months	10th year
Second molars	20 months	24 months	11th or 12th year

cleaning however many teeth he has to establish good dental hygiene habits.

Caring for your baby's teeth begins as soon as the first tooth erupts. After feeding, wipe its surface with a damp washcloth. As more teeth come in, introduce your child to brushing. Brushing techniques differ for primary teeth and permanent teeth. They differ, too, from one dentist to another, even from one year to the next, as dental research discloses the long-range effects of various dental-hygiene programs. Unless your dentist advises otherwise, here is a method suitable for brushing the primary teeth.

How to Clean and Rinse the Primary Teeth

1. Choose a child-size toothbrush with soft nylon bristles and use a fluoride toothpaste.

2. Using a circular motion, gently scrub a few teeth at a time. Be sure to include the gums and don't neglect the inner surfaces of the teeth. Let your child take over, if he likes.

3. Follow up with the "swish-and-swallow" rinsing technique. Teach your toddler to take a sip of water and swish it around the teeth before swallowing. You don't use toothpaste with swish-and-swallow, just water. Repeated three times, this is highly effective in removing bacteria and makes up for a small child's less-than-perfect tooth-brushing skills. The child can spit out the rinse as well, but swallowing it is easier for most small children. And swish and swallow works well after meals when spitting isn't possible.

Supplement nightly toothbrushings with the swish-and-swallow cleaning method after meals and snacks.

The point of all this effort is to remove plaque. Plaque is a sticky, whitish film composed of bacteria, saliva, and food debris that clings to tooth surfaces causing tooth decay and gum disease. It's hard to see plaque and tell where it's accumulating, and it is even harder to convince children that it's there. That's when disclosing tablets come in handy. These tablets (available at the drugstore) contain a harmless dye that turns plaque bright red and then fades within a matter of hours.

Testing for Plaque

Explain to your child that this test will show which parts of her mouth need extra brushing.

1. Give her one disclosing tablet and tell her to chew on it for about a minute, swish it around in her mouth, and then spit it out. (It's harmless if she happens to swallow it.)

2. Areas where plaque has accumulated, usually between teeth and at the gum line, will be bright red. These are the areas that need extra attention. Be sure to reassure your child that the color will be gone by morning.

3. Repeat the test nightly until the disclosing tablets reveal little or no plaque on your child's teeth. Stubborn deposits may have to be removed using a rubber-tipped probe that usually can be found next to the toothbrushes in the drugstore. Then, regular professional cleanings as your dentist recommends should keep the baby teeth as clean as possible.

Fluoride Treatment

Many dentists believe that fluoride treatments promote sound teeth. Fluoride is available in four forms: in fluoride toothpastes, in fluoride treatments given by the dentist, in the water supply of some communities, and by prescription. Ask your dentist if the local water supply is fluoridated. (This can occur naturally or it may be added to the water.)

If it is not, the dentist or pediatrician (if your baby is still too young to go to the dentist) may prescribe fluoride supplements, available in either chewable tablets, in vitamins, or as a liquid that may be dropped directly into the mouth or mixed with cereal, fruit juice, or other food. Dosage depends on the age of the child and the concentration of fluoride in the water supply. So don't use the same prescription for more than one child without the dentist's or doctor's approval. And if you move, check with your new dentist or pediatrician before continuing with fluoride supplements.

Monitoring the Primary Molars and the First Permanent Molars

Before your child loses his first primary tooth, the first permanent molars will probably have erupted. Also called the six-year molars because they usually appear at around age six, these teeth come in just beyond the primary molars. There is one on either side of each jaw for a total of four. These molars guide the placement of subsequent teeth.

The first permanent molars usually erupt between ages five and seven. Well before they appear, however, you should keep an eye on the primary molars.

CHECKING THE PRIMARY MOLARS. Just as the first permanent molars guide the placement of subsequent teeth, so do the primary molars guide

in the permanent six-year molars. By age five at the latest, check to see that all eight primary molars (two at either end of the jaw, top and bottom) are in view and are positioned properly. If any appear crooked, consult the dentist.

WATCHING FOR THE FIRST PERMANENT MOLARS. Beginning around age five, periodically check the gum tissue just beyond the primary molars for signs of the first permanent molars. When these molars break through, check their placement and positioning. If any of these appear crooked to you, bring this to the attention of your child's dentist immediately.

Occasionally, one of these teeth erupts through the gum, leaving a flap of tissue where food particles can collect. When this happens, the gums can become sore and infected. In such cases, the dentist may choose to cut away this flap of tissue.

Once the six-year molars are in, the rest of the permanent teeth should emerge pretty uneventfully.

Nursing Bottle Caries

Most parents are aware that sweets and other foods with a high sugar content promote cavities (caries). By far the greatest threat to a baby's teeth, however, comes from another source—the bedtime bottle.

Many parents routinely put a baby to bed with a bottle of juice or milk. Juice or milk are not in themselves harmful to teeth, though they do contain some sugar. The problem lies in the method of feeding. Baby sucks, nods off, and the liquid pools in his mouth, bathing the teeth in sugar for hours at a time. It's like giving your baby an all-day sucker every night.

The cumulative effect of this practice is widespread decay of the teeth, especially in the upper jaw. This characteristic pattern of decay is so recognizable and so common in toddlers that it has acquired a term of its own—*nursing bottle caries* (*caries* means tooth decay).

The solution, of course, is not to put a baby to bed with a bottle of juice or milk. A bottle of water is good at bedtime or naptime, but give other drinks only in a cup.

Checking for Cavities

Supplement your child's regular visits to the dentist by checking your child's teeth yourself. In addition to your penlight and tongue blade, you will need a dental mirror. An inexpensive plastic dental mirror can be purchased at most drugstores.

Have your child brush her teeth and rinse thoroughly with warm water. Run warm water over your dental mirror to keep it from fogging up during your examination.

Use your penlight in coordination with your dental mirror. Hold your dental mirror behind the tooth surface you wish to observe, shine the penlight into the mirror, and let it reflect its light onto the tooth. This way you can examine both easy-to-see and hidden surfaces. Also use the mirror to help keep the tongue out of your way. You should be able to master the technique with a bit of practice.

Examine each tooth carefully and methodically for evidence of decay. Cavities are most commonly found between the teeth, at the gum line, and in the grooves on the tops of the teeth. A cavity is seen as a small hole, usually stained a blackish color. (The hole on the outside, by the way, is much smaller than the hole being made on the inside.)

Be sure not to miss any tooth surface in your examination. If you find a suspicious-looking spot, make a note of it and report it to the dentist.

Tooth Loss Due to Injury

Small children commonly bump their teeth on furniture and receive inadvertent blows to the mouth

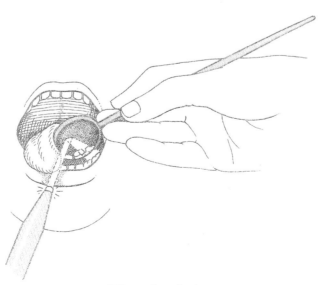

Using a dental mirror

in the course of play. Sometimes the damage is obvious—a chipped tooth or a tooth knocked out. The dentist should see these, of course. Other times, the damage may not be at all obvious at first. If the nerve inside the tooth has been damaged, the tooth will die gradually, over a period of days. You cannot prevent such mishaps, aside from making your home and play areas as baby-safe as possible, but you can recognize the signs of nerve damage that may result from a blow to the mouth.

If a permanent tooth is knocked out and can be found intact *with* the root, rinse it off, save it in a small amount of milk, and bring it to the dentist within an hour. If the roots and tooth are not broken, sometimes the tooth can be rerooted in the gum.

Recognizing Nerve Damage in a Tooth

Discoloration in a tooth or in two adjacent teeth that were white and healthy looking just a short time ago is a strong indicator of nerve damage. In such cases the tooth begins to die, changing color in the process. This color change can range from gray to yellow to brown or black. If you notice this kind of isolated color change in a recently healthy tooth, treat it as a dental emergency.

The dentist probably will not opt to do extensive work in order to save one of the primary teeth. Most likely, he will insert a spacer device that maintains the gap and keeps the other teeth in their proper position.

CHAPTER 9

HOW TO EXAMINE YOUR BABY'S BONES AND MUSCLES

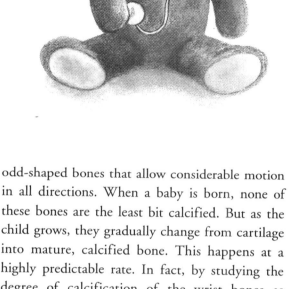

There are more than two hundred bones in the body, linked by joints of various kinds, and manipulated by innumerable muscles. Muscles are attached to bones by stiff cords of fibrous tissue called tendons, and bones are attached to one another by dense, fibrous bands called ligaments. Together, these five components—bones, muscles, tendons, joints, ligaments—make up what is known as the musculoskeletal system.

Your Child's Bones

Between the fifth and the twelfth week after conception, miniature structures having the shape and the appearance of adult bones, but composed of cartilage, can be discerned in the developing embryo. Soon the cartilage begins to be replaced by bone, and the body's structural girders lengthen and harden.

Some parts of a newborn's skeleton are still composed almost entirely of unossified bone tissue. The wrist, for example, contains two rows of odd-shaped bones that allow considerable motion in all directions. When a baby is born, none of these bones are the least bit calcified. But as the child grows, they gradually change from cartilage into mature, calcified bone. This happens at a highly predictable rate. In fact, by studying the degree of calcification of the wrist bones as revealed by x-rays, doctors can determine a child's physiologic age with an accuracy of between three and six months—valuable information when treating a child with growth retardation.

On the other hand, the long bones of the arms and legs—which must bear weight from an early age—are substantially ossified at birth, but not without allowing for future growth. This is provided for by the epiphyseal plates at either end of the long bones. These are slices, or plates, of cartilage from which new growth can arise. When the epiphyseal plates finally harden, between the fourteenth and twenty-fifth years, further growth ceases.

To a parent, the epiphyseal plates should be of more than passing interest, since injuries to the

111

long bones that affect these areas can seriously interfere with normal growth.

The Muscles and Tendons

Bones do not act independently, but rather are acted upon by the muscles that control them. Muscles, as noted previously, are attached to bones at either end of their length by stiff cords of fibrous tissue called tendons. The attachments are generally made across a joint, with one end of the muscle attached to a bone on one side of the joint and the other end of the muscle attached along a bone on the other side of the joint.

When a muscle contracts, one of the bones will move about the joint in the direction of the muscle pull. To get that bone back to its original position requires that the first muscle relax while another pulls from the opposite direction. Thus, it takes a minimum of two muscles to move a bone around a joint and bring it back again.

In practice, however, a great many muscles are involved in moving any part of the body in any direction. It is this interaction of many muscles pulling in slightly different directions that allows the body to make subtle movements.

Most of these movements are beyond a baby's ability at birth. Gradually, however, the randomly flailing legs and the reflexive clasping and unclasping of fists yield to finer and more controlled movements. With practice, your baby soon learns to hold a bottle, pick up a raisin, walk, and make all the other breathtakingly complex movements that most of us take for granted.

The Joints and Ligaments

There are different kinds of joints, allowing for different kinds of movements. The elbow is a hinge joint; it can fold up or down, like the lid of a box. The knee is another hinge joint. The hip, on the other hand, and the shoulder, too, are ball-and-socket joints. The knob, or ball, at the end of the long bones is free to rotate nearly 180 degrees in the rounded-out socket of the joint. Other joints, like the cartilaginous discs between the spinal vertebrae, allow only limited movement.

Tough bands of fibrous tissue, called ligaments, encase each joint, binding adjacent bones together and forming a fibrous capsule lined with lubricating membranes. Muscles and tendons, bones and ligaments all come into play at the various joints to provide a wide range and variety of body movement.

Your Baby's Musculoskeletal System

A baby's musculoskeletal system has all the same parts as an adult's, but it is not exactly the same. The spine has yet to acquire its adult curvature, for example, or the foot its arch. And different kinds of problems tend to crop up as well. A hip joint may be too shallow, the feet may turn in or turn out more than they should, and so on. You need to know, then, what is special about your baby's musculoskeletal system, and what to be on the lookout for. Here is a selective look at areas of special concern.

Your Baby's Head

Four bones cover the entire top of the head: the front down to the eyes is covered by the frontal bone; the sides, extending well around toward the back, are each covered by one of the two parietal bones; and the back, right down to the neck, is covered by the occipital bone.

In an adult, all of these bones are tightly knit together. In an infant, however, the skull must allow for growth. It does this by maintaining gaps between the unossified edges of these bones. These soft edges are connected to one another by bands of connective tissue along suture lines.

How to Feel the Suture Lines

Use the tip of your index finger to feel the suture lines, which are like cracks between the bones of the skull (see the diagram, "Location of the fontanels," in Chapter 1).

1. First examine one of the two most prominent sutures, the frontal suture, which sweeps across the front part of the top of the head.

2. Next use your index finger to feel the other prominent suture, the sagittal suture, which is the line down the middle of the top of the head.

3. Lastly, feel the occipital suture at the back of the head.

In the newborn, the sutures may feel slightly open or occasionally overriding. This latter phenomenon is particularly common along the sagittal suture, where, because of pressure on the skull during birth, one bone slips over another just a bit. This is felt as a step when you run your hand across the top of the baby's head. Both open sutures and overriding sutures should not be cause for concern in the first week or two of life. Overriding sutures usually straighten themselves out within a week or two at most.

Rarely, the sutures of the headbones will already be fused at birth. This is usually, but not always, associated with other deformities of the head and is felt as a ridge along the top of the head. If you find such a ridge, bring it to your doctor's attention immediately.

At the point where two suture lines intersect, there is a gap called a fontanel.

How to Feel the Fontanels

The fontanels can be felt as soft spots at the intersection of the suture lines.

1. First feel the largest fontanel, the anterior, or front, fontanel, which is a diamond-shaped spot at the junction of the frontal and sagittal sutures, on top of the head. At birth, this fontanel measures about two and a half inches from side to side, and about an inch in length.

2. If you follow the sagittal suture line down and back toward the neck, you will find the posterior, or rear, fontanel, a triangular area where the sagittal suture meets the occipital suture.

Normally, the posterior fontanel is closed by age three months. The serrated edges of the suture lines have begun to knit together by six months, and by twenty months, the anterior fontanel has been replaced by bone.

The Spinal Column

Structurally, the spinal column is composed of segments of bone called vertebrae. A typical vertebra consists of a round, flat bone and a pair of bony arches that meet to form a circular enclosure at one end. Three bony spurs project off this end of the vertebra; you can feel the middle one, called the spinous process, as one of the bony bumps going down the back.

The individual vertebrae (there are twenty-four of them) are stacked one on top of another to form a canal down the vertebral column. This is the bony fortress that houses the spinal cord linking the brain with the rest of the body. Nerves branch off the spinal cord at various points through openings in the vertebrae.

In between the vertebrae, there are walled capsules of cartilage containing a resilient, jellylike substance. These are the discs.

Each vertebra is connected to the one above and below by ligaments that serve the same purpose here as they do at other joints—that is, they maintain adjacent bones in the proper relationship.

The vertebral column is held erect with the support of three basic muscle groups that, together, act like guy wires—each exerts the precise amount of pull needed to hold the spinal column erect.

The Neck

The first vertebra at the top of the spinal column is attached directly to the base of the skull. This one, plus the next six, are the cervical vertebrae that make up the bones of the neck.

Wryneck, or twisted neck deformities, sometimes occur when one of the neck muscles is injured during birth. As a result, the chin is rotated to the side opposite the affected neck muscle. The head is tilted toward the side of the injury. It is sometimes possible to feel a lump in one of the neck muscles. This represents the area of injury.

In mild cases, passive stretching exercises are usually quite effective. But if the deformity has not been corrected by these exercises within the first year of life, surgical correction will be necessary. Because of possible involvement of the spinal column, all children born with a twisted neck should be treated by a physician.

Children, like adults, sometimes develop a stiff or twisted neck following a mild respiratory infection. A simple neck collar may add to the child's comfort, but the condition usually resolves itself within a few days. Acetaminophen and heat will generally make the child more comfortable. A mild injury may also lead to a temporary stiff or twisted neck. These should always be brought to the attention of a doctor because of the possibility of injury to the spinal column.

The Back

Your main concern in examining your child's back is to observe its curvature. Curvature refers to the normal curves that develop naturally in the spinal column.

The back of a newborn infant has a C-shaped curve that gives young babies a round-backed look. As the baby learns to hold up his head, however, a new curve is acquired where the cervical vertebrae of the neck flex to support the head. Later, when the child is walking, a second, inward curve develops lower down, just over the buttocks. This curve adjusts the body's center of gravity so that the spinal column can support the weight of the upper body. The result is the typical double-S curve, most pronounced and easily seen in the flexible back of a young gymnast.

Problems arise when either of these curves becomes exaggerated, or when a side-to-side (lateral) curvature develops.

Exaggerated curves of the spine are usually remarked upon as "poor posture" and typically develop in early adolescence, a time when skeletal growth outpaces muscle growth. Special exercises that strengthen shoulder and abdominal muscles usually correct the problem.

Posture is rarely a problem in children under six. However, any child who appears to be gradually developing abnormal posture should be checked for scoliosis. Scoliosis is a twisting of the spine so that when the child is inspected from behind, standing upright, the spine appears to be curved to one side, rather than straight up and down.

Scoliosis is most common after the age of eight or ten, and is about four to five times more common in girls than boys. There is, however, a type of scoliosis that occurs in younger children, between the ages of two and four. This condition is far less common in the United States than the type of scoliosis that occurs in older children.

How to Test for Scoliosis

1. Have the child stand up straight with her back bared to just below the waist. The little knobby protrusions that run down the center of the back (the spinous processes) should line up in a perfectly vertical column that doesn't deviate the least bit from side to side.

   If you have trouble locating the spinous processes, have the child bend forward slightly from the waist. This makes the bony knobs more prominent. Then, using a black felt-tip pen, make a little dot on the skin directly over each spinous process. Have the child stand straight again. The little dots should form an absolutely straight line in the center of the back.

2. A dropped shoulder is another sign of scoliosis. With the child standing as before, check to see that one shoulder does not drop lower than the other.

3. Have the child stand with her legs spread slightly apart and bend foward slowly at the waist, keeping her knees straight and letting her arms hang down in front. As the the upper body drops downward, watch closely from

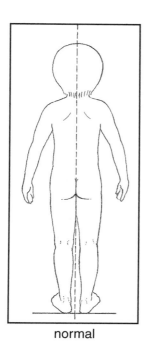
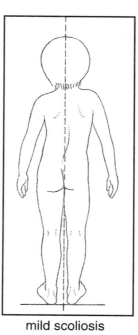
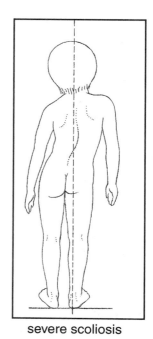

| normal | mild scoliosis | severe scoliosis |

Detecting scoliosis

behind to see if one side of the torso is higher than the other at any time. Both sides should remain equal.

4. You may be able to detect scoliosis in its very earliest stages by recognizing an uneven development of the back muscles. Have the child lie on the floor, stomach down, with her hands behind her neck. Hold her legs down and and ask her to raise her upper body so that the chest just clears the floor. Hold this position for a moment or two. **(Caution: Do not do this exercise with any child who has been experiencing back pain or other back problems.)** Lay your hand, palm down, on the muscles of the back first on one side and then the other. The muscles should be equally developed on both sides of the spine. Uneven development may indicate incipient scoliosis.

The Hips

One of the most common of all skeletal abnormalities, occurring about once in every five hundred births, is congenital hip dysplasia. The word dysplasia means an abnormality in development. In this case, it is the socket of the hip joint that is abnormally developed.

Normally, the head of the femur, the upper leg bone, fits into the socket of the pelvis, or hip bone. In some infants, for reasons that are not known, this socket does not develop properly and is too shallow to hold the ball of the femur in place. Consequently, when pressure is exerted at the joint, the ball of the femur tends to slip upward out of the socket, resulting in partial or complete dislocation of the hip. Testing for congenital hip dysplasia is covered in Chapter 1, "The First Examination of Your Newborn Baby." Treatment

is simple if begun early, and it will prevent lifelong deformity.

The Feet and Legs

The lower leg contains two bones—the tibia and the fibula. The ankle, like the wrist, contains a number of odd-shaped bones that give the foot mobility in all directions. The rounded prominences on either side of the ankle, called the malleoli, are actually flared-out ends of the lower leg bones.

The feet, like the hands, contain five long bones extending out to each toe, and the toes contain either two or three bones each, depending on the toe. In addition, the foot contains a bone at the heel, the calcaneus, which transmits the body's weight to the ground.

There are a number of minor deformities of the lower leg and foot that parents should be aware of: bowleg, knock-knee, tibial or femoral torsion, flat feet, metatarsus varus, and pronated ankles. Descriptions of how to detect each of these conditions follow. A more serious deformity, clubfoot, is also discussed.

Bowleggedness

Bowleg is the common name given to legs that curve outward from the hips. This is normal from infancy to about two years of age or so. When a baby starts walking, the lower back and leg muscles become better developed and the legs gradually straighten.

How to Check for Bowleggedness

1. Have your child stand with his feet together and his shoes off. Measure the space between

the knees. If this space is greater than one inch, then bowleggedness is present.

2. Any bowing of the legs beyond age two-and-a-half, bowing that is increasing instead of decreasing, or bowing that is greater in one leg than in the other, should be brought to the attention of your doctor.

Knock-Knee

Knock-knee is the opposite of bowleg. In this condition, the legs curve outward from the knees. Like bowleg, knock-knee is normally present at a certain age—in this case, from about two to three-and-a-half years. Extreme knock-knee, however, or knock-knee that persists into childhood, should be evaluated by the doctor.

How to Check for Knock-Knee

1. Have the child stand straight with her shoes off.

2. Measure the distance between the malleoli—the rounded prominences of the ankles.

3. This measurement should normally be less than one inch. If this space is greater than one inch, the child is said to be knock-kneed.

Tibial Torsion

The tibia is the main bone of the lower leg, and torsion simply means twisting. Thus, tibial torsion is a twisting of the lower leg.

A baby's legs are normally bowed at birth and remain bowed until he starts walking. Tibial

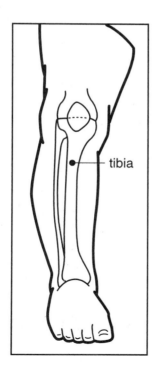
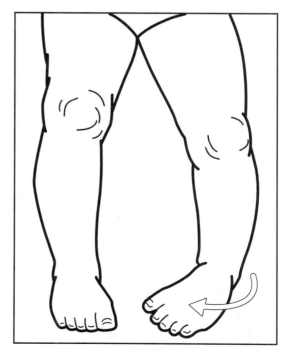

Tibial torsion

torsion adds an inward twist to the normal bowing effect that causes the inner sole of the foot, where the arch will be, to turn sharply inward and upward toward the body. While the condition can occur in both legs, the left leg is more frequently affected than the right.

How to Check for Tibial Torsion

There are two methods for checking if your child has tibial torsion.

1. Observe the position of the baby's legs when he is lying on his back. Normally, if you bend the baby's knees and bring them together, the feet will point straight upward. If tibial torsion is present, however, the foot of the affected leg will point inward when the knees are brought together.

2. Place the baby face down on the floor, or hold him in your arms, facing you. Tibial torsion in one leg will cause both feet to point in the same direction, instead of pointing outward in opposite directions.

Femoral Torsion

A condition similar to tibial torsion in children beyond the age of two or three is usually based on internal rotation of the femur rather than the tibia, so it is called femoral torsion. It almost always affects both legs, causing them to turn inward, limiting the normal range of motion.

How to Check for Femoral Torsion

1. Have the child lie on her back with her legs fully extended and her feet pointing up.

2. Normally, you should be able to rotate each foot about fifteen degrees inward and about sixty degrees outward. In a child with femoral torsion, however, you will barely be able to turn the feet outward at all.

3. Inward rotation, on the other hand, extends a full ninety degrees so that the inside of the foot, from heel to big toe, can be laid down flat.

Both tibial torsion and femoral torsion should be brought to the attention of your doctor. But many physicians now feel that treatment with special shoes or braces has little effect and that the condition will usually correct itself by age eight or ten. Exercises such as bicycle riding, ballet dancing, and skating can be helpful in correcting this kind of minor abnormality.

Flat Feet

Flat-looking feet are normal in babies. The arch in the foot does not develop for several years. If you are concerned about your child's flat feet, make the following observations.

How to Assess Flat Feet

1. Have the child sit or lie comfortably so you can easily inspect the bottoms of the feet.

2. Place the feet in a neutral position. Then check to be sure that the foot moves freely, both upward and downward.

3. Next, look and see if the foot is in an arched configuration. If you are able to move the foot freely, both upward and downward, and if there appears to be a normal arch when the child is not bearing weight, the child will, in all likelihood, eventually develop a normal arch.

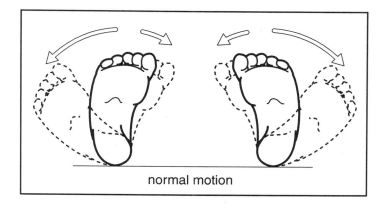

normal motion

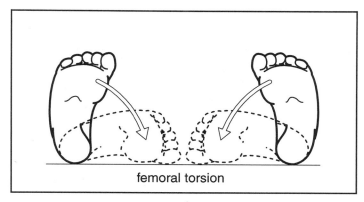

femoral torsion

Femoral torsion

If there is no arch even when the child is not weight bearing or if the foot is not freely movable, both upward and downward, consult your doctor.

In many cases, no treatment is necessary unless the child is having leg pains due to flat feet. In this case an orthopedic shoe with a special arch may be helpful. Shoe arch inserts should not be used without medical advice.

Metatarsus Varus

The metatarsal bones of the feet connect the heel bone with the toe bones. Metatarsus varus is a bending inward of the upper half of the foot. The condition is usually apparent at birth, and can affect one or both feet. This condition is easy to recognize if you examine the soles of your baby's feet.

How to Recognize Metatarsus Varus

1. Normally, a baby's feet should be straight from heel to toe, so that if you draw a straight line up from the center of the heel, it will pass through the third toe, dividing the foot in half lengthwise.

2. In metatarsus varus, however, the foot curves inward like a large apostrophe, so that a line starting from the center of the heel would go through the two smallest toes at the outside of

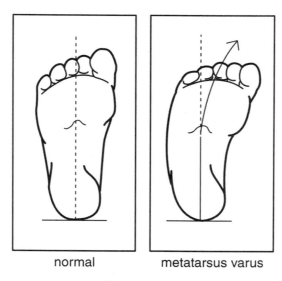

normal   metatarsus varus

Metatarsus varus

the foot. In this case, you would have to draw a curved line to connect the center of the heel and the third toe.

If the foot is somewhat flexible, the deformity can be corrected by frequent, gentle manipulation, which a parent can do under a doctor's direction. If the deformity is more rigid, short-term plaster casting may be necessary. Corrective shoes are expensive and rarely do much good. Complete correction of this minor deformity can be expected.

Pronated Ankles

Pronated means turned downward, and this is what pronated ankles do. In this condition, both ankles turn inward toward the ground. The problem becomes readily apparent after the child starts walking, at which time parents notice that she seems to have no arch. Flat feet in young children, as noted earlier, is generally not cause for concern. Pronated ankles, on the other hand, are definitely abnormal and should be seen by a doctor.

How to Recognize Pronated Ankles

1. Look at your child's legs from behind while she is standing. Draw an imaginary line starting at the center of the heel and going straight up the leg.

2. This line should bisect the middle of the heel, the heel cord, the center of the ankle, and the center of the knee.

3. If the child has pronated ankles, your imaginary line from heel to knee will pass outside the ankle joint. Or, to put it another way, the line would have to swerve inward at the ankle to bisect heel, ankle, and knee.

A child with pronated ankles will wear out a pair of shoes along the inside edge of the soles and heels. The upper part of the shoes will also be broken down along the inner side because of the excessive pressure exerted by the pronated ankles. This condition is generally corrected with special shoes, arch supports, and other devices prescribed by your doctor.

Clubfoot

A clubfoot is an uncommon but serious deformity in which one or both feet point downward and inward, with varying degrees of severity.

This condition is obvious at birth and corrective manipulation and the use of plaster casts should begin immediately. Otherwise, the foot tends to become rigid within a matter of days. Once the foot has been corrected to its normal configuration, some kind of bracing is usually necessary to prevent recurrence. Even with prompt treatment, about half the children born with clubfeet eventually require some kind of surgical intervention.

Injuries That Affect the Bones, Muscles, and Joints

At some time during most children's lives, some kind of trauma occurs to the musculoskeletal system. Bones may be broken, muscles strained, joint ligaments sprained.

Many people are confused by the terminology used to describe such injuries. Knowing these terms will help you to understand and deal with the kind of problems they refer to, so please take time to familiarize yourself with the terms in the following glossary.

A Glossary of Musculoskeletal Injuries

Fracture. The word *fracture* is simply a medical term for a break. It is important to keep in mind that a broken bone and a fracture are the same thing.

Strain. A strain is a tiny tear in a muscle or tendon (tendons attach muscles to bones).

Contusion. A contusion is damage caused by a blow that injures a muscle or the soft tissues under the skin, causing bleeding within the muscle. A black-and-blue mark is a manifestation of a contusion.

Sprain. A sprain is a more severe injury that occurs when a ligament (ligaments bind bones together across a joint) is torn or stretched.

Dislocation. When the stress on a ligament is so great that it knocks either opposing bone ends or a bone end and its socket out of position, the injury is called a dislocation.

Bone Fractures

There are different kinds of fractures: bends, greenstick fractures, buckle fractures, and complete fractures.

A child's bones, particularly the smaller of the two bones of the forearm and lower leg, can bend as much as forty-five degrees before breaking. When severely bent, the bone will straighten out slowly but will leave a deformity. A bone stressed in this way is called, appropriately enough, a bend.

A bone bent beyond its limit is apt to break part way through, like a green twig, and is thus called a greenstick fracture.

When a bone is compressed and creates a bump or bulge at the site of the break, it is called a buckle fracture.

A complete fracture is one that divides the bone into two parts.

How to Recognize a Broken Bone

Diagnosing a broken bone is not all that difficult, though you may get precious little information from the child himself. He is apt to be either too young to communicate well, crying too hard to talk much, or reluctant to disclose the forbidden activities that led to the broken bone. A broken bone typically exhibits the following four symptoms:

1. *Pain.* The area around the broken bone will be very painful.

2. *Loss of normal function.* The child will be unable to bear any weight at all in the case of a broken leg or be able to use a broken arm.

3. *Muscular rigidity.* The muscles in the area of the break will be hard and tensed. This is because the muscles contract to "splint" the injured area.

4. *Swelling and discoloration.* Finally, a generalized swelling engulfs the entire area, and accompanying contusions will appear as black-blue-purplish discolorations.

Because children are so susceptible to injuries, parents should have a good working knowledge of basic first aid. Many good books are available, and we recommend that you have one in your home. Basic courses in first aid are offered frequently by the American Red Cross, YMCA, and other agencies. When there is a course in your community, take it.

But even if you are quite confident of your first aid skills, call for professional help when you suspect a fracture. Keep the child off a broken leg, and immobilize a fractured arm. Don't move the child if you suspect a back or neck injury. Fractures of the upper arm bone (the humerus) are particularly dangerous and tend to occur most often in the three-year-old to six-year-old age group. The swelling may be severe and the main artery to the arm is often very near the point of the break. Avoid

manipulating an arm with a break in the humerus. Don't try to remove clothing, for example.

A child with a broken arm will often hold the arm close to his body and his hand low on his stomach, with the elbow just slightly bent. This is a natural splinting position, and if you can immobilize the arm easily in this position (a large towel bound around the body and the arm will do it), the child will be more comfortable while waiting for medical attention. If you have to do any major manipulating to get an injured part into a comfortable position, it's best to leave it alone until professional help arrives.

Many children fracture the clavicle, or collar bone. The child will complain of shoulder pain and will have difficulty raising the affected arm. Collar bone fractures are usually treated by the doctor with a figure-eight splint, which simply pulls the shoulders back. A lump often develops on the bone during the healing process, but this disappears within a year or so.

Children's bones heal rapidly with good medical management. You can expect a young child to recover from a fracture within four to six weeks, and most of the time physical therapy isn't needed. Children tend to work at restoring normal function themselves, but a doctor's advice must govern in this regard.

Muscle Injuries

Common muscle injuries include contusions, strains, and muscle cramps.

Treatment for both contusions and strains consists of prompt application of an ice pack for fifteen minutes or so at intervals throughout the day. After ice treatments for the first twenty-four to thirty-six hours, apply hot packs for twenty minutes, three or four times a day to speed the healing process. Be certain the hot pack is no warmer than you can comfortably tolerate yourself. **Caution: You must be absolutely certain before undertaking treatment of what you believe to be a contusion or strain that you are dealing with that type of injury and not a fracture.**

Muscle cramps may occur in children, particularly after strenuous exercise. A good treatment is to have the child take a hot bath for thirty minutes, twice a day, while you help him to exercise and massage the affected muscles underwater. Give your child appropriate doses of acetaminophen or ibuprofen for the pain.

About a third of all children, at some time, have nighttime muscle cramps in their feet or calf muscles. These can be quite painful and will usually waken the child from sleep. During the attack, pull the foot and toe upward as far as possible to break the spasm. Gently massage the hard, cramped area. The attack should pass within a few minutes. Future attacks can sometimes be prevented by daily stretching exercises, such as toe touches. Quinine is also used in the treatment of nighttime muscle cramps, and a glass of quinine water before bedtime may help if your child is experiencing this annoying problem frequently.

Joint Injuries

The most common joint injuries fall into two categories: sprains and dislocations.

A sprain is a joint injury where the ligaments holding the joint together are seriously stretched or even torn. Ankle sprains, for example, typically happen when there is an unexpected twist of the ankle. Sprains, particularly those in which there is actual tearing of the ligaments, should not be taken lightly. A serious sprain with one or more torn ligaments can be a much more bothersome long-term

injury than a clean bone fracture. Many doctors will apply a plaster cast to sprains to help the ligament heal in a normal position. Therefore, even if you are quite certain that nothing is broken, have a physician check any child who sustains a sprain injury.

When the stress on the ligaments is so severe that bones are wrenched out of position, the joint is said to be dislocated. This kind of injury causes a deformity that is readily apparent. Other symptoms are pain and loss of function of the affected joint.

One of the most common dislocations in small children involves the head of the radial bone (one of the two bones of the lower arm) at the elbow joint. This is sometimes referred to as "nursemaid's elbow." It can happen when an adult lifts or pulls an infant or toddler along by one hand. If the child's arm is already fully extended, an adult's rough upward jerk can literally wrench the radial bone out of position. Once this dislocation occurs, the child will not bend the elbow and will be in considerable pain. This can happen when a child tries to go in one direction and the adult, in an effort to restrain him, pulls with a jerk in another direction.

The child will complain of pain, not necessarily in the elbow. She may say, "My wrist hurts," for example, and will refuse to use the arm for anything, letting it hang by her side.

The dislocation can usually be reduced (that is, pushed or put back in place) with a simple manipulation by the doctor. Prevent this injury by avoiding rough arm play and by not pulling or swinging your young child by one arm.

Other dislocations to ankles, knees, hips, shoulders, and fingers can be much more severe— skating and skiing accidents, rough-and-tumble play, or falls from trees can all cause dislocations— and all must be given professional care.

Finger Injuries

Children's fingers are frequently injured. They are jammed in doors, hit with hammers, bruised, smashed, or crushed in any of a number of ways. Take a child with injured fingers to the doctor

- if she is not able to open and close any finger normally at all joints

- if there is a large, open cut since it may require stitches

- if there is so much dirt in the wound that you can't scrub it all out

- if there is bleeding under the fingernail

Bleeding under the fingernail can be particularly painful for a number of days. A physician can almost immediately relieve the pain by making a small hole in the nail to allow the blood to drain out.

Any time a finger is injured and doesn't seem to require medical attention, soak it in ice water for the next hour. Take the finger out of the water every fifteen minutes or so for a few minutes to prevent frostbite. This treatment will cut down the swelling and make it easier to determine the extent of the injury. Torn nails should be trimmed and filed with an emery board to prevent them from catching on clothing and bed sheets.

A good way to prevent little fingers from getting caught in car doors is to command, "Simon says, 'Hands up.'" When all hands are raised, it is probably safe to shut the car doors.

Diseases That Affect the Musculoskeletal System

Osteomyelitis

Osteomyelitis is a bacterial infection of one or more bones. The invading bacteria may have entered the body via a penetrating wound, a bone fracture that breaks through the skin, burns that become infected, or from infections that cause such illnesses as tonsillitis, middle ear infections, and abscessed teeth, among others.

It is most common in children between five and fourteen years of age, and occurs more often in boys than in girls. The long bones of the arms and legs are the usual sites, and the knee area is a common site as well.

In infants, the symptoms may be subtle. The baby may simply be irritable, have diarrhea, or fail to feed properly. In such cases, the diagnosis is difficult to make. Symptoms are much more pronounced in older children, however. There is usually severe tenderness and swelling over the affected bony area. The child is likely to have a high fever, a rapid pulse, and no appetite. Laboratory studies reveal a strikingly elevated white blood count.

Osteomyelitis requires prompt and aggressive therapy in a hospital setting. Any child with a limb that is so painful he does not wish to move it, and who acts generally ill as well, should be taken to the doctor immediately.

Joint Swellings

Joint swellings are never normal in children. They are due either to trauma—an accident or injury— or to an infection in the joint, which can be extremely serious and must receive prompt medical attention.

In infants, infections of the hip joint are the most common, particularly if there has been some difficulty in the newborn period requiring the placement of a small tube into one of the umbilical blood vessels. Limited motion of one leg compared to the other should alert you to this possibility.

Prompt treatment is necessary to prevent serious damage to the joint. Recovery is usually excellent if treatment is begun within twenty-four hours of the development of the illness. If treatment is delayed, serious damage to the joint and to the nearby growth plate of the long bone may result.

Toxic Synovitis

Children between three and ten years sometimes develop a pain in the hip that causes them to limp. It is more common in boys than in girls and is commonly caused by an irritation of the lining of the joint capsule. The condition is called toxic synovitis, and it often follows a mild respiratory illness. Treatment usually consists of simple bed rest, and the problem clears in about a week. However, the condition can be confused with a much rarer bacterial infection of the joint capsule, so it is wise to consult a physician to confirm the diagnosis.

Juvenile Rheumatoid Arthritis

Stiffness, swelling, tenderness, and loss of motion in one or more joints are a few of the many symptoms of arthritis, a condition that, unfortunately, is not all that uncommon in children.

There are different forms of juvenile rheumatoid arthritis, or JRA. One form occurs most commonly in children under four and starts as a salmon pink, flat rash together with inflamed joints and enlarged liver and spleen. One or more joints may be involved.

In children between nine and twelve years, the disease is more like that of adult arthritis, with chronic swelling and pain affecting many joints both large and small. A third pattern in older children involves only one or two joints, usually the large, weight-bearing joints. Swelling may be more pronounced than pain, and there may be little fever, fatigue, or other generalized symptoms. Children with the latter two kinds of arthritis may also develop eye problems and should visit an ophthalmologist every six months.

No home treatments or folk remedies for arthritis should be attempted for children. Obtain prompt and expert medical advice in order to limit the ravages of this disease as much as possible.

Lumps

Lumps that seem to be associated with a bone—especially near the ends of long bones of the arms and legs—should always be viewed with suspicion and reported to your doctor. Such lumps can indicate the existence of a bone tumor. Lumps or unusual hard spots in muscles should also be reported for the same reason.

Muscle Problems

Disorders of the muscles (that are not caused by injuries) are considerably less common than disorders of the bones and joints. One of the major problems is distinguishing whether the disorder lies in the muscle itself or in the nerves that stimulate the muscle into action.

Muscle problems generally present themselves as clumsiness; fatigue when walking, running, or climbing stairs; diminished control of face muscles or other muscles; drooping eyelids; or, in infants, a generalized floppiness. This kind of generalized muscle problem, medically termed dystrophies and myotonias, are relatively uncommon and usually inherited. Generalized muscle weaknesses should be evaluated by a specialist.

CHAPTER 10

HOW TO TEST YOUR BABY'S NERVOUS SYSTEM

Within days of conception, specialized cells within the embryo group themselves along three longitudinal structures. One of these, called the notochord, is a sturdy rod destined to become the backbone. The other two, on either side of the notochord, are hollow tubes. The one in front develops into the digestive system. The other, lying behind the notochord, is the embryonic precursor of your baby's nervous system. Three little bumps at the front end of this neural tube, as it is called, swell to become the lobes of the brain. The remainder become the spinal cord. Eventually, the nerves stream out from the spinal cord to all parts of the body.

The result, at birth, is the marvelously complex nervous system, responsible for processing information about the body and its environment, and dictating appropriate instructions in response.

Different parts of the nervous system have different responsibilities. Knowing which part plays what role in your baby's body will give you a better understanding of the tests which follow.

The Anatomy of the Brain

The brain consists of three segments: the cerebrum, the cerebellum, and the brain stem. The cerebrum is by far the largest of the three segments. It consists of the two great lobes of the brain, called the cerebral hemispheres, which lie next to each other and fill most of the skull.

Deep inside these cerebral hemispheres are open spaces called ventricles—a vestige of the neural tube's hollow origin—filled with a watery substance called cerebral spinal fluid. This fluid also fills the space surrounding the spinal cord. When the doctor performs a spinal puncture or tap, he withdraws a small sample of this fluid for analysis.

The cerebral hemispheres control the higher functions such as reason, speech, memory, smell, taste, vision, and movement. One hemisphere is always dominant over the other. If your baby turns out to be right-handed, his left hemisphere is probably dominant, and vice versa.

127

The cerebellum sits below the rear half of the cerebral hemispheres. It controls functions we don't usually think much about, such as balance, coordination, and kinesthesia. Kinesthesia is the ability to know where a part of the body is located and what it is doing without looking at it.

The third segment of the brain is the brain stem. This rounded knob is actually the upper end of the spinal cord. The brain stem controls what are referred to as vegetative functions. These functions include—among others—breathing and heartbeat, which continue whether or not your baby is awake or asleep, aware of them or unaware of them.

The Spinal Cord

The spinal cord originates at the brain stem and runs down the protective bony canal formed by the spinal vertebrae. It is sometimes thought of simply as a cable, or trunkline, of nerves connecting the brain with the rest of the body, but it is actually much more than this. The spinal cord carries out some functions that might ordinarily be thought of as brain functions. For example, a knee-jerk reflex is a spinal-cord function. This reflex is called an arc because the nerves that receive the tap on the knee send the signal to the spinal cord, the signal is processed right there, and the message directing the muscle to jerk is sent right back.

The Nerves

Nerves transmit information from all parts of the body to the brain and spinal cord and relay orders back. Thirty-one pairs of major nerve bundles branch off from the spinal cord, and a special set of nerves, called the cranial nerves, emanate directly from the base of the brain. There are twelve pairs of cranial nerves (one nerve from each pair for the right side of the body and one for the left) controlling important functions such as taste, smell, vision, and eye movement, to name just a few.

Testing Your Baby's Nervous System

Despite its breathtaking complexity, a basic evaluation of your baby's nervous system is carried out using very simple equipment. Some tests require a ball of cotton or a little rubber hammer. Others use some common flavor extracts. A small toy is sometimes called for, and a few tests are done by observation alone. Unlike other medical specialists, neurologists rely less on x-rays, complicated tests, and elaborate equipment than on close observation and careful reasoning.

Obviously, it takes years of training and experience to detect subtle symptoms of neurologic disorders. Still, it is possible to perform a fairly complete evaluation of your child's nervous system yourself. The simple tests and observations described below should help you spot abnormalities that should be brought to the attention of your doctor and will also tell you when things are normal and working well.

Most of the tests in this chapter are for older babies and young children because the nervous system is still rather immature at birth. Tests for newborns are described in Chapter 1. The nervous system continues to mature through the childhood years so that some of the tests that follow are age-dependent—meaning only a child of a certain age can be expected to have acquired a particular skill. This age, moreover, may vary from one child to another. Thus, an age range, rather than a specific age, is the usual guideline, as you will see.

A basic evaluation of the nervous system should check cerebellar functioning, the cranial nerves, the deep tendon reflexes, muscle strength, coordination, and, in older children, speech and reasoning.

Cerebellar Functioning

The cerebellum is the part of the brain that controls balance and coordination, called motor skills because they involve movement. Your baby's gradual mastery of movements is followed in some detail in Chapter 14, "Tracking and Testing Your Child's Growth and Development." Two kinds of motor movements are presented in that chapter: the gross motor movements, such as crawling, standing, walking, and running; and the fine motor movements, such as picking up small objects, buttoning clothes, or tying shoes. If your child is achieving these developmental milestones at an appropriate age—as described in that chapter—then the cerebellum is functioning normally. If, on the other hand, your child lags in achieving these developmental milestones, you should point this out to the doctor.

By the time a child is ready for kindergarten—say, age four or five—he should be able to perform balance and coordination tests.

How to Test Balance and Coordination

A cooperative three- or four-year-old should be able to do the following tests. Demonstrate each maneuver first and let your child practice a bit.

1. *Finger-to-nose test.* Have your child extend her arm out in front of her, then bring it in and touch her nose with her forefinger. Have her do this first with her eyes open, and a second time with her eyes closed. It's okay for a preschooler to miss by a few inches.

2. *Romberg Test.* Have your child close his eyes and stand with his heels together. He should be able to stand up straight without falling or leaning to one side.

If your school-age child has difficulty performing these tests with the eyes open, it may be an indication of poor coordination. Difficulty performing these tests with eyes closed suggests poor position sense. Have a doctor evaluate either of these findings.

The Cranial Nerves

Twelve pairs of cranial nerves emanate from the base of the brain. Some are responsible for one particular function, such as sight or hearing; others control more than one function. (Cranial nerves are usually numbered with roman numerals, which is what we will do here.)

I. THE OLFACTORY NERVE. The first cranial nerve is called the olfactory nerve. This pair of nerves connects with the nasal turbinates in the back of the nose and controls your baby's sense of smell.

How to Test the Olfactory Nerve

1. You will need two or three common flavor extracts from the supermarket. Choose flavors that your child can readily recognize—peppermint, cherry, or orange, for example. Make sure he knows the names of these familiar scents.

2. Test each nostril separately. Have the child close one nostril by holding a forefinger against it. Then, one by one, unscrew the little bottles and ask your child to take a whiff and tell you what he smells. If he can read, be sure to cover the label with your hand. Repeat the test for the other nostril.

3. If the child can correctly identify the scents both times, then his first cranial nerve is said to be intact.

II. THE OPTIC NERVE. The second cranial nerve, the optic nerve, controls your baby's sense of sight. This nerve bundle leads out from the back of each eyeball, crosses its partner a little way back, and makes its way toward the rear part of the brain. The vision tests described in Chapter 6 are actually tests of the second cranial nerve. If your child can pass those then his second cranial nerve is in good working order.

III, IV, AND VI. THE NERVES THAT CONTROL EYE MOVEMENT. The third, fourth, and sixth cranial nerves govern the muscles that control eye movement. One allows your child to gaze up, another to gaze down, and the other to look from side to side, without moving her head. They all work together in a coordinated fashion, so one test will suffice to check all three.

How to Test the Eye-Movement Nerves

1. Hold a bright toy about two feet in front of the child's eyes. Instruct her not to move her head, but to follow the toy with her eyes. A very young child may not understand these directions, so have a partner hold her head gently.

2. Move the toy from side to side and up and down, and watch how the child follows it with her eyes. If both eyes follow the object in all directions and in coordination with each other, then the nerves that control eye movement are functioning correctly.

V. THE TRIGEMINAL NERVE. The fifth cranial nerve, called the trigeminal because it has three branches, controls (among other things) the chewing muscles and the sensation of light touch over the face.

How to Test the Trigeminal Nerve

1. Check the muscles used in chewing by instructing your child to bite down hard and then open again, two or three times. Muscle strength should appear equal on both sides of the jaw.

2. You will need a wisp of cotton to check light touch sensation over the face. Instruct the child to close his eyes and tell you when he feels the wisp of cotton touch his face. Lightly touch the skin on the lower half of the face in several places. An inability to sense two or more touches may be an abnormal finding and should be called to the attention of your doctor.

VII. THE FACIAL NERVE. The seventh cranial nerve is the facial nerve. Two of its most important functions are the sensation of taste on the front two-thirds of the tongue and the control of the muscles of expression.

How to Test the Facial Nerve

1. Make your baby smile by playing peekaboo, tickling her lightly, or some such game. Her facial expressions should appear equal on both sides of the face. A crooked smile, in which one side of the mouth crinkles naturally while the other side remains relatively expressionless, is a telltale sign of a seventh-nerve disorder.

2. To test taste sensation, prepare separate solutions of sweet-, sour-, and bitter-tasting liquids in little cups. Sugar water or honey will do for the sweet taste, a concentrated solution of instant coffee for the bitter (one teaspoon of instant coffee in two tablespoons of hot water and let it cool), and white vinegar for the sour. Before testing, go over the difference between bitter and sour with your child.

3. Instruct your child to stick out her tongue. Take a cotton-tipped swab, dip it in one of the solutions and apply it to one side of the tongue. Rinse with plain water between tests. An older child should be able to identify each solution correctly and separately on each side of the tongue.

4. When testing a very young child, it is sufficient to observe a pleased expression in response to the sweet substance and a grimace in reaction to the bitter and sour solutions.

VIII. THE AUDITORY NERVE. The eighth cranial nerve, the auditory nerve, hooks up with the inner ear and has two functions. The first is hearing. If your baby can pass the hearing tests presented in Chapter 5, then that aspect of eighth-nerve function is normal.

Another part of the auditory nerve leads to the semicircular canals of the inner ear, which affect balance and position sense. The tests described previously in this chapter under "Cerebellar Functioning" are also good tests of the eighth cranial nerve. Disorders of this nerve are usually associated with dizzy spells and some degree of hearing loss.

IX. THE GLOSSOPHARYNGEAL NERVE. The ninth, tenth, eleventh, and twelfth cranial nerves are interrelated in a number of ways. For instance, the ninth and tenth nerves share responsibility for the gag reflex. Disorders of the ninth and tenth cranial nerves may also affect the eleventh and twelfth, and vice versa. Within this network of shared functions, however, there are functions controlled largely by one nerve. These lend themselves nicely to home testing.

The prefix *glosso-* refers to the tongue, and *pharyngeal* to the pharynx, or the throat. The ninth cranial nerve, then, affects the tongue and throat. More specifically, it controls taste sensation for the back third of the tongue and stimulates the gag reflex.

How to Test the Glossopharyngeal Nerve

1. To stimulate the gag reflex in a child old enough to cooperate, instruct the child to open his mouth wide and say ah-ah-h.

2. Lightly touch far back on the tongue or the back wall of the throat with a tongue depressor. The child should gag. Do this gently. You don't want to elicit a major reaction.

X. THE VAGUS NERVE. The tenth cranial nerve, called the vagus, has a great many functions. Branches of the vagus are involved in the secretion of stomach acid. Parts of the vagus control some of the muscles in the roof of the mouth that help form normal speech sounds. The vagus is also involved in swallowing. If your baby has been swallowing her food and milk without difficulty, then the vagus nerve is functioning as it should.

XI. THE SPINAL ACCESSORY NERVE. The eleventh cranial nerve controls certain muscles in the shoulders. You can easily check this aspect of eleventh-nerve function in any child old enough to shrug his shoulders.

How to Test the Spinal Accessory Nerve

1. Have your child raise both shoulders as if shrugging them, but instead of lowering them, keep them raised.

2. Place your hands on both his shoulders and push downward while the child tries to keep the shoulders elevated. Exert an equal amount of force on both sides. Both the child's shoulders should resist with equal strength.

XII. THE HYPOGLOSSAL NERVE. The twelfth and last of the cranial nerves is the hypoglossal, which controls the muscles of the tongue.

How to Test the Hypoglossal Nerve

1. Have your child stick out her tongue. It should protrude straight out, though a slight deviation to one side is not uncommon.

2. Have her move it in all directions—up, down, and to each side. Demonstrate if necessary.

3. Check muscle strength by placing your tongue blade against one side of the tongue and instructing the child to move it away.

4. Repeat the test on the other side. Muscle strength should appear about equal on both sides of the tongue.

5. *For a baby,* simply observe how she uses her tongue. A functioning tongue is used well in such activities as nursing and babbling, par-

ticularly the consonant sounds such as da-da and ta-ta.

The Deep Tendon Reflexes

A reflex is an automatic response dictated by the nervous system. A newborn baby is a bundle of reflexes, many of which you can test yourself as described in Chapter 1. These primitive reflexes of the newborn gradually subside, however, and by four months, only those persist that remain through life. Among these are the deep tendon reflexes.

Deep tendon reflex testing is usually done using a small, rubber-headed hammer. The head of this hammer may be either triangular in shape or cylindrical with rounded ends. If you wish to purchase a reflex hammer, they are available at medical supply stores and are relatively inexpensive. Actually, almost any little weight on the end of a short arm will do as well, such as a rubber spatula or a wooden mixing spoon.

There are four deep tendon reflexes that can be tested in children. Two of them are arm reflexes and two are leg reflexes. You can test three of them easily.

How to Test the Knee-Jerk Reflex

The knee-jerk reflex, the most familiar of all neurologic tests, checks nerves serving the lower leg.

1. Sit the child on a chair or on a partner's lap so that his legs swing freely from the knees without touching the floor.

2. Locate the kneecap with your fingers. This is the rounded bone that sits right over the knee.

3. Next, locate the bony prominence just a little below the kneecap. This is the top end of the

large bone of the lower leg. You should be able to feel a stiff cord running in the short space between the bottom of the kneecap and the top of the leg bone. Mark an X over this cord using a felt-tip pen.

4. It is easier to elicit a reflex when the child is not too intent upon what you are doing. Distract the child by having him hook his hands together, hold them up in front of his chest, and pull outward as hard as he can while keeping his hands hooked. This increase in general muscle tone often strengthens the knee-jerk response as well as distracting the child.

5. Using your small rubber hammer or other appropriate instrument, briskly tap the knee at the point you have marked. Remember, it is a tap you deliver and not a blow. If the test is done correctly, the lower leg will immediately give a little jerk upward.

6. Repeat the test on the other knee.

The normal response in this test is extremely variable. Some children will show a very active response, while others will demonstrate a weak knee-jerk reflex. The most important observation, however, is not the strength of the response, but the equality of response in both legs. Both legs should jerk upward by about the same amount. A knee-jerk response that is substantially more active on one side than on the other should be evaluated by the doctor.

How to Test the Ankle-Jerk Reflex

The ankle-jerk reflex tests the nerve bundle running down the back of the lower leg, which serves the foot.

1. Have the child sit on the edge of a chair or table or in your partner's lap so that her legs dangle freely.

2. Just above the heel bone, running up the back of the leg, locate a very strong, fibrous cord. This is the Achilles tendon.

3. Mark an X with your felt-tip pen over this tendon at about the level of the ankle.

4. Lightly grasp the front half of your child's foot in one hand and press upward ever so slightly.

5. Using your other hand, tap the Achilles tendon with your reflex hammer. It takes a moderately hard tap to elicit a response, but you don't want to deliver a hurtful blow. Try tapping your own Achilles tendon first to get the feel of the test. If the test is done correctly, the foot should jerk downward just a bit.

6. Repeat the test on the other ankle.

As with the knee-jerk response, the Achilles tendon reflex should be about equal on both sides.

How to Test the Biceps Reflex

The biceps is the big muscle on the front part of the upper arm. When you bend your arm, you are using your biceps muscle. The biceps attaches to the lower arm, across the elbow joint, by a tendon that passes down the center of the inside of the elbow.

1. First locate your child's biceps tendon: feel just alongside the hollow that forms on the front of the arm when his arm is slightly bent. In this hollow, just off center, you will feel a strong cord, which is the biceps tendon. Mark an X with your felt-tip pen over this tendon.

2. Facing your child, hold his partially bent elbow in your hand and press your thumb gently on the tendon right over the X you have made. Support your child's forearm in such a way that it can be totally relaxed.

3. Using your reflex hammer, strike sharply on the thumb you are holding over the X mark. If the test is done correctly, you should feel the tendon tighten under your thumb an instant after the thumb is struck. The child's arm may also give a little jerk upward.

4. Repeat the test on the other arm.

As with the other reflex tests, the biceps reflex should feel about the same on both sides.

Reflexes that are equal from side to side but apparently more brisk in the legs than in the arms are usually not a cause for concern. It is only when the responses are unequal on the two sides that a professional opinion should be sought.

There are many other nerve responses that you can't test, of course. Every body function has its own system of nerves that serves it. So any marked change in body control or function should be considered from a neurologic viewpoint if some other, more obvious, explanation is lacking.

Recognizing Coma in Your Child

Coma is a sleeplike state from which the child cannot be aroused or can be aroused only with great difficulty. It is probably the most dramatic and serious sign of severe central nervous system problems.

Early stages of coma might be described as "stupor" or "confusion." The child looks awake and his eyes are open, but he does not act awake—

that is, he does not follow objects or persons with his eyes, or does so only slowly, and he does not speak. He has difficulty following even simple directions, is apt to be disoriented in time and place, and has trouble identifying people.

In more pronounced stages of coma, the child appears to be sleeping but cannot be aroused from it. He will react to loud sounds, bright lights, or pain by trying to withdraw from these things. He commonly makes sudden movements with his arms or legs. His speech, if any, will not make sense, and he will probably lack bowel or bladder control.

If your child shows any such symptoms, call your emergency medical service for transportation to the emergency room and then notify your doctor.

Try to collect your thoughts so you can describe as clearly as possible the events leading up to the coma. There are many possible causes. Poisoning is a common cause of coma in children, resulting from ingesting medicines, alcohol, or any number of other substances in the house; and from inhaling volatile substances such as those found in glues and cements, or from carbon monoxide in gas stoves or automobile exhausts. (Become familiar with home safety procedures outlined in Chapter 15.) Some substances, such as drugs and inhalants, act very quickly, while others, such as heavy metals, take days or even weeks to produce ill effects.

Trauma (injury) from a fall or from being hit can also cause coma, as can childhood diabetes and liver and kidney failure. (Diabetes is discussed at length in Chapter 12, which deals with the endocrine system.) Finally, children who have had an epileptic seizure may be difficult or impossible to arouse for several hours after (though this is not a coma).

Bleeding in the brain can occur without trauma. On rare occasions, a small aneurysm may develop in an artery in the brain. Known as a berry aneurysm, it is a swelling or ballooning of an artery wall that bursts, allowing bleeding into the brain. It is a condition seen mostly in adults but occasionally happens to children.

A doctor presented with a comatose child, without any other information, will have no idea which of this rather large number of possible causes to investigate first. She is, therefore, totally dependent on the medical history you provide to help her decide where to start. The following are some clues to the causes of coma you should look for.

1. *An open bottle of pills.* A partially empty, still open bottle of pills is a good clue to medicine intoxication. Take the bottle with any remaining pills along with you to the hospital.

2. *A fever or earache.* If your baby or child has had a fever for some days and has suddenly become worse, particularly if there has also been an earache, this is a clue to the doctor that the baby may have meningitis.

3. *Trauma.* If the child has fallen or received a blow to the head recently, this is, of course, a very important piece of information.

4. *Weight loss and poor health.* Children with liver or kidney failure, or with developing diabetes, have often lost weight and develop a look of less than full health before lapsing into a coma.

It is vital for the doctor to know all of these things. Time is extremely important when treating meningitis, intoxications, and, of course, bleeding within the skull. The doctor needs all the help she can get in terms of the child's health history, which she can learn only from you.

Reye's Syndrome

Reye's syndrome is a poorly understood condition that affects the central nervous system. It seems to appear at about the time a viral illness, such as chicken pox or the flu, is resolving. One theory links the use of aspirin for a viral illness with the development of Reye's syndrome, which is why aspirin should be avoided in treating childhood illness. In any event, the child suddenly seems much sicker with fever, vomiting, irrational behavior, progressive stupor, and, finally, coma.

Though not common, the condition is severe. It worsens rapidly and requires prompt expert treatment. This treatment is best accomplished in a large teaching hospital rather than in a community hospital.

With prompt treatment, at least three-quarters of the children with Reye's syndrome are now surviving, many of them without ill effects. Call the doctor immediately if a child who is recovering from the flu or chicken pox seems to be having a relapse and is becoming stuporous.

Meningitis

Infections of the central nervous system can also cause coma. One such infection is meningitis, an infection of the coverings of the brain and spinal cord, caused either by bacteria or a virus. Viral meningitis is a far less threatening disease than bacterial meningitis. Several varieties of bacteria can cause meningitis and both the severity of the disease and the long-term outcome depend at least in part on the specific type of bacteria with which your child is infected. Early recognition of the disease and aggressive treatment is essential. If you suspect your child has meningitis, get him to an emergency room and notify your doctor.

A child with meningitis will act sick, have a fever, and have a stiff neck, caused by spasm in the neck muscles, to the extent that he is unable to touch his chin to his chest. He won't want to turn his head. As time goes on the child becomes stuporous and will not respond to you as quickly as a few hours before.

In one particularly severe form of meningitis, children develop tiny, pinhead-size red spots on their bodies that are caused by tiny blood vessels under the skin that have broken. **This is a medical emergency.**

Convulsions

Convulsions (also called seizures) are among the most common—and frightening—of nervous system disorders. Years ago, people who had convulsive disorders, such as epilepsy, were social outcasts, and children who suffered convulsions were often hidden from society. The truth is, however, that the majority of children with convulsive disorders have perfectly normal intelligence and, with proper medication, can lead normal lives in every way.

The term *epilepsy* refers to a chronic, or recurring, pattern of convulsions. There are many types of convulsions, the four most common being febrile, grand mal, petit mal, and psychomotor seizures.

Febrile Convulsions

Febrile means fever-related, and this type of convulsion occurs most commonly between the ages of six months and four years. It is triggered by a sudden rise in body temperature. Most febrile convulsions occur when the baby's temperature suddenly shoots up to 102°F or more, and they usually strike during the rapid rise rather than after—which means that they tend to come on unexpectedly. They are sometimes the first sign of a cold or flu. Tonsillitis and other infections of the throat, together with a middle ear infection, are the most common associated illnesses.

When evaluating a convulsion the doctor will want to know if there has been any illness associated with the event, such as flu or an earache. If this is the case, and this is a first or isolated incident, he will probably prescribe fever-reducing agents and perhaps cool baths before searching for deeper neurological problems.

Although febrile convulsions are frightening, they have little long-term significance. Most children with febrile convulsions have a normal brain wave pattern and outgrow the tendency by age six or so.

Grand Mal Seizures

Grand mal seizures are not related to fever. They can strike at any age and usually occur without warning. Some children, however, seem to have a sense of foreboding, also called an "aura," that an attack is about to occur. This might take the form of a visual hallucination ("See the stars, Mommy!"), or it could be a hallucination involving odors. It may consist simply of a "funny feeling" that prompts the child to start running for his mother or father when an attack is imminent.

The child who suffers his first grand mal seizure should be taken to see the doctor immediately. The brain wave tracing is usually abnormal in such children. Although very brief seizures of this kind appear to have no permanent ill effects on the child, it is thought that some prolonged seizures temporarily interrupt the blood supply to the brain and may cause some damage. For this reason, it is important to control grand mal seizures with drug therapy. Skilled pediatric neurologists have found that they are able to achieve excellent seizure control in most children.

Recognizing either a febrile or a grand mal convulsion is not hard, but it can be a frightening event the first time you see one if you don't know what to expect or what to do.

How to Recognize a Febrile Convulsion or a Grand Mal Seizure

1. The episode begins with a sudden loss of consciousness, sometimes announced by a piercing cry. The child falls to the floor as if she has been knocked down by some unseen force.

2. The eyes roll up, the teeth clench, and the body is wracked by rhythmic, twitching movements. She may breathe heavily, froth at the mouth a bit, and lose control of bladder and bowel. The convulsion may last anywhere from a few seconds to a few minutes.

3. Afterward, the child seems confused, may feel achy and, if left alone, usually sleeps for several hours.

There is nothing you can do during a convulsion to stop it. Just stay with the child and see that she doesn't injure herself. If she is not in bed, ease her to the floor. Loosen any tight clothing.

Petit Mal Seizures

Petit mal seizures are also known as "absence attacks." They consist of brief lapses of consciousness—perhaps five to ten seconds—during which the child seems to stare vacantly into space. The eyelids may blink rapidly, and there may be facial twitches, grimaces, or slight hand movements. This type of seizure is considerably rarer than the grand mal type and is pretty much limited to children over the age of three or four.

Psychomotor Seizures

These are similar to petit mal. They consist of vague staring; facial, tongue, or swallowing movements; sometimes throaty, unintelligible utterances; and often complicated, automatic movements such as walking, running, or kicking.

It is important for parents to be aware of these last two types of seizures because they are sometimes mistaken for behavior that the child can control. The momentary lapses of consciousness may be dismissed as "daydreaming," and the repetitive twitches as calculated attempts to "get on a parent's nerves." If your child displays this kind of gesturing, facial grimacing, or automatic movements, coupled with a "faraway look" about him, you should recognize this as a possible seizure disorder and consult your doctor.

Breath-Holding Spells

Breath-holding spells are often mistaken for epileptic seizures, but they are actually exaggerated tantrums triggered by frustration. Typically the child will start off by crying violently and screaming, and then will suddenly hold her breath. She will continue to hold her breath until she begins to turn blue, and eventually she loses consciousness. Occasionally, at this point, the child will have an extremely brief seizure lasting only a few seconds. This is unusual, however. Once the child is unconscious, she loses voluntary control over breathing and begins breathing normally again. Consciousness soon returns, and, because of the drama of the situation, the child often finds herself surrounded by the attention she was seeking.

Unless the child hits her head or otherwise injures herself when she falls, these spells are not dangerous. They are strictly an emotional display, and treatment with medicines is of no benefit. Children with frequent breath-holding spells should be seen by a physician to be certain there is no underlying disorder. Once the diagnosis has been definitely established, however, it is wise to pay as little attention as possible to the child during one of these episodes. If breath holding fails to produce the desired effect for the child, she is more likely to stop.

Headaches

Headaches afflict children, though they are less common than in adults. In infants, your only clues are apt to be prolonged irritability, crying, and head rolling. Children too young to tell you where it hurts will be fussy and will resist attempts to handle or amuse them.

If your child develops a headache, the first thing to do is to be sure he has not received a blow to the head. Look for bruises and black-and-blue marks. If the child is old enough to talk, ask him if he has hit his head or if he has recently been hit in the head.

The most common kind of headache, in children just as in adults, is the simple tension headache. It can be caused by unusual excitement or by stress in the child's life. The tension headache is a constant dull pain that covers the entire forehead on both sides. Often the neck muscles are also achy.

Treatment with rest and a child-appropriate dose of acetaminophen usually takes care of the immediate problem. Contact your doctor if a headache lasts for more than twelve hours or if it becomes worse after two to three hours. For the long run, you should investigate what it is that is causing stress and tension in your child's life.

You should call the doctor if your child has a headache plus any of the following problems:

- Vision problems such as blurring or double vision
- Unsteadiness while standing
- Confusion or not acting normally
- Difficulty speaking or is difficult to arouse from sleep
- Vomiting
- Can't touch the chin to the chest while lying down.

Occasionally, headaches are caused by eye problems, but this is far less common than is generally believed. Children as young as four can get migraine headaches, though these are difficult to diagnose unless the child is able to describe the symptoms. The migraine attack is usually pounding, throbbing, or pulsating in character. It may involve one side of the head or both, or simply the front part, or just behind the eyes. Nausea, stomach discomfort, or vomiting are commonly associated with these headaches. Children with migraine headaches tend to prefer darkened rooms. Rest plus acetaminophen will help relieve symptoms, but any child with a migraine-type headache should be seen by a physician. There are a number of medicines available for treatment, and occasionally they can prevent migraine attacks.

Brain Tumors

Cancers of all types are the second most frequent cause of death in children over the age of one. (Accidents are number one.) Of the various kinds of cancers, brain tumors are second only to leukemia. Specific diagnosis of brain tumors is often delayed by six months or more, and it is therefore important for parents to be aware of some of the early symptoms.

- Frequent and worsening headaches that seem to be most painful when the child wakes up in the morning

- Vomiting that is not associated with nausea or feeding

- In infants, bulging of the fontanels and widening of skull sutures

- Staggering or difficulty walking in a child who has already mastered these skills

Other symptoms that can be caused by a brain tumor include speech difficulties, vision problems, severe weight loss, seizures, and difficulty using one arm or one leg. All of these should alert parents to the possibility that something is seriously wrong. One particular type of tumor that can often be satisfactorily treated is associated with the presence of five or more café au lait spots scattered somewhere on the body (café au lait spots are described in Chapter 2, "How to Examine Your Baby's Skin").

Tics

Tics are quick, repetitive, spasmodic movements that can be controlled at will. That is to say, if the child has a tic and you tell her to stop, she will be able to stop the spasm easily—for the moment, anyway. The most common types of tics are facial twitches, grimaces, and blinking. Twisting and throwing movements of the arms and trunk are also common.

Tics are most common in children between the ages of nine and thirteen, but they can occur much earlier. Unlike the facial twitches and quick movements that can accompany a seizure, tics have an emotional basis and are usually associated with an underlying psychologic problem. Often, if a family pays a great deal of attention to a particular tic, it will increase in intensity and become more elaborate or be replaced by another, even more distracting tic. Emotional therapy is usually effective.

Paralysis

Because of widespread immunization, polio and the paralysis it causes are very uncommon now. There are, unfortunately, other causes of paralytic disease in children. The most common of these, Guillain-Barre syndrome (infectious polyneuritis), starts off as a weakness in both feet and legs, rapidly working its way upward to involve the trunk, arms, and face. In severe cases, the respiratory muscles are affected as well. Rapid medical attention is always necessary. Fortunately, the paralysis is not permanent and, although the child may be unable to move for a number of weeks, the majority of children recover completely. A few are left with some residual weakness.

Another type of limb and body paralysis is caused by tick bites. Ticks are small, bloodsucking insects that attach themselves to the skin. The first symptom is usually irritability, followed some twelve to twenty-four hours later by paralysis, which starts with the legs and moves upward.

The diagnosis of this type of paralysis rests entirely on finding the tick. If you find any insect attached to your child's body, remove it using rubbing alcohol, being sure to get the head, which is often embedded in the skin. Removal of the tick is followed by rapid improvement and total recovery. But if your child develops any symptoms of illness, see the doctor.

Behavioral and Perceptual Difficulties

A wide array of difficulties in learning and behaving often beset children who are normal in every other way, meet most developmental milestones, and may even be of above-average intelligence. In some, however, language development may be slightly delayed. A short attention span and a variety of learning disabilities may manifest themselves. Hyperactivity and overexcitability can be major problems.

These difficulties have accumulated a broad array of labels that are constantly changing, mostly because there are so many variables from child to child and because the people studying these problems are still without real answers to the cause of the problems. And there is no real agreement about broad solutions that can work for every child. Attention deficit disorder (ADD), hyperactivity, and behavioral difficulties are among the labels attached to children who may be angry, aggressive, can't sit still, and have a short attention span. While this describes the behavior of every child from time to time, some children seem continually to be in these difficult moods.

Learning disability, dyslexia, and perceptual problems are labels used for children who may perceive letters and words differently, or who find it difficult to cope with number systems and calculations in the way they are set up for the rest of us. While these children can be labeled "dumb" by their peers, they may be remarkable in other ways, in the arts and athletics for example.

Depression and anxiety often accompany these conditions because the child experiences so many frustrations in learning and social interactions. These children can present major problems for their parents and teachers, and they require all the patience and inventiveness a parent can muster.

Treatment is largely supportive and psychologic. Children will need remedial tutoring, which is best not done by the parents but by someone else with a calm and patient nature, who is experienced in dealing with such children. Behavior modification programs under the guidance of a psychologist are sometimes helpful. Drugs must be used sparingly and with care. They cannot be used as a substitute for a strong and aggressive behavioral program. Dealing with these problems requires a great deal of patience and the understanding that the condition will continue for years.

Some schools have teachers who are trained to work with children who have behavioral, perception, or learning disabilities, and most states require that schools have personnel who can evaluate children as young as three so that special programs can be set up for them as early as possible. However, a teacher may have so many children to look after, your child will get minimal attention at best. If at all possible, these children should receive competent help outside of school special-education programs. Your pediatrician will be able to offer guidance in finding appropriate treatment.

Keep in mind, however, that no child is a good-natured cherub who is eager to learn all of the time, any more than the adults in the family are. So before you attach a label to a child, be sure that the problem you perceive is a real one and has been evaluated by a competent professional.

Chapter 11

Checking on Baby's Bottom and Urinary System

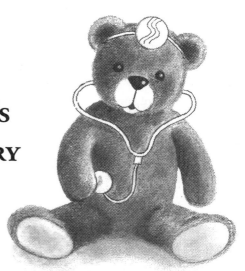

Baby's urinary system makes itself known most obviously in the way it keeps you busy changing diapers. Urine output, however, besides keeping you from getting bored with nothing to do, furnishes important insights into your baby's health.

Many jokes are made about stool watching and urine watching, but this is one area of function the doctor rarely sees and parents always do, so the first signs of anything being amiss in either of these departments will invariably be seen by parents. Urinary tract infections and such diseases as diabetes, which affect urine composition and output, often produce very subtle symptoms. Only a careful observer is likely to become suspicious that something is wrong. So it pays to be informed.

The Urinary System and How It Works

The urinary system rids the body of excess fluids, salts, and nitrogen products. This is accomplished in the kidneys, which are located high against the back wall of the abdomen, one on either side of the spine. You can't feel them, but to identify the approximate location of the kidneys, find your lowest ribs and follow these back until you reach the spinal column. The kidneys lie in the angles, on each side, formed by the spinal column and the lower margin of the bottom rib. Two tubes—the ureters—one from each kidney, carry urine from the kidneys to the bladder. The bladder is located in the lowest part of the abdomen behind the pubic bone in adults. It's a bit higher in babies and descends slowly throughout childhood to its adult position. When full, the top of the bladder expands upward and it is possible to feel this soft, balloon-like structure rising above the pubic bone.

Finally, the urethra runs from the bladder to the outside of the body. This tube is longer in boys, having to make its way through the penis, and shorter in girls, ending between the labial folds, just forward from the vaginal opening. Because the urethra is short in girls, they have many more problems with urinary infections than boys.

141

The kidneys are highly specialized, highly complicated filters, filled with thousands of small structures called nephrons. Each nephron consists of what seems to be a crumpled-up ball of tiny blood vessels, surrounded by a membrane. This membrane comes together to form a tube that winds around a bit and then enters a common collecting system in the central portion of the kidney. The tubes of the collecting system come together to form the ureters.

A portion of the fluid content of the blood passes through the filters of the nephrons. Protein components of the blood are held back by the filtering membranes while water and dissolved salts pass through. But much of the salt and water is reabsorbed in a very selective way. If the body has too much water or too much of a specific kind of salt, less will be reabsorbed. If the body is low on salts and fluid, the looped tubes will reabsorb almost all the water and salt passing through. On the average, less than 1 percent of all the fluid filtered by the kidneys ever makes it to the bladder as urine.

Observing Urinary Function and Signs of Dysfunction

Careful observation and an intimate knowledge of your baby's normals are especially important in detecting problems with urinary function. Symptoms are often vague—baby is wetting more or less than usual, he is vaguely lethargic or fatigued, he develops puffiness that seems at first like healthy weight gain. On the other hand, there may be alarming symptoms, which turn out to be quite innocuous. You may be frightened to see pink urine until you remember that the baby had beets for supper. There may be alarming pain in the kidney area that results from hard play and disappears the next day. Following are things to think about in evaluating your child's urinary function.

Quantity of Fluid Intake and Output

A baby quickly establishes a pattern of feeding. And you soon know how often you have to change wet diapers. If a baby suddenly becomes an insatiable feeder, or an older child exhibits unusual thirst without good reason, something could be wrong. If you suddenly notice there are many more diaper changes, more trips to the bathroom, or many fewer, once again something could be wrong. A child who is urinating frequently because she is developing diabetes will pass relatively large amounts of urine (see Chapter 12, "What You Should Know About Your Baby's Endocrine Glands and Hormones").

Patterns of Urination

Urination should be effortless and the stream, strong and steady. Signs of developing problems include obvious discomfort, difficulty starting, narrowing of the stream, dripping of small quantities when there is an urge to go, frequent dribblings, loss of control in a child who has already established good control (day or night). Some symptoms, such as reoccurrence of bed wetting, may result from a new stress or worry in the child's life, but check with your doctor in any event.

Appearance of the Urine

Color of urine can vary for perfectly harmless reasons. Urine is normally clear and some shade of light yellow. It is sterile and slightly acid. Foods and drugs can change the color, however, so think what the child has been eating before you become alarmed over a color change. Blood in the urine is always abnormal. But beets can cause red urine in some children. Brown or tea-colored urine can be a sign of disease, but rhubarb, cascara, and a number of medicines can darken urine. Aspirin and sulfa drugs create shades of yellow; riboflavin, B-complex vitamins, and yeast can turn the urine green. Persistently foul-smelling urine should be investigated, though eating asparagus will produce an offensive odor in some people.

Some General Symptoms

Urinary problems sometimes follow a flulike illness. Symptoms may include fatigue or lethargy even though the child is not otherwise ill. Persistent lower abdominal pain or other discomfort signaled by squirming or irritability should be checked, though these can have causes other than urinary problems. Puffiness of the eyes, ankles, feet, and other extremities—especially occurring in the morning—should always be investigated. Sometimes this swelling seems like normal baby growth or healthy weight gain, so you have to be alert for changes you know intuitively are not right. Unusual weight gain or loss should always be checked. Pallor is another symptom that sometimes accompanies urinary problems. Persistent pain in the back in the kidney area, particularly on one side, should be investigated. A change in blood pressure can be an important clue to kidney disease. (Chapter 3 describes the procedure for taking blood pressure.)

All this is not as confusing as it seems if you keep in mind that changes—especially unexplainable changes—are what you should watch for. If you think you notice a disturbing symptom, consider the whole range of your child's recent activities and behavior: foods and medicines taken; accidents or injuries that may have occurred; recent illness, stress, or worry the child may be experiencing.

Sometimes a child will experience a spasm of the valve at the opening of the urethra. After not urinating for more than a usual interval, he feels the need to go but is unable to pass any urine at all. Try sitting your child comfortably in warm water. Chat quietly, tell a story, and encourage relaxation. Encourage the child to urinate directly into the water. Your encouragement and the relaxing effect of the warm water often do the trick, but if this doesn't work, see a doctor immediately.

Urinary Tract Infections

Urinary tract infections are the most common cause of abnormally frequent urination in children, boys and girls, but they affect girls far more frequently than they do boys. Organisms from many sources have easy access to the bladder and beyond through the short, straight urethra of young girls. The longer route through the male penis is more difficult for invading bacteria to negotiate. Tight clothing, soiled diapers, local infections, detergent soaps, even bath water are more hazardous to a girl's urinary tract than to a boy's.

Depending on where the infection lies, urinary tract difficulties are given different names: urethritis is an inflammation of the urethra; cystitis is an inflammation that has reached the bladder; ureteritis is an inflammation of the ureters leading from the kidneys to the bladder; and pyelonephritis is an inflammation of the kidneys.

Frequency of urination and some pain or burning is the most usual early sign of a urinary tract infection. Typically, the child will complain that she has to pass urine, but when she tries, she passes only a small amount. As the infection works its way higher toward the kidneys, there may be some elevation of temperature, chills, and others of the symptoms mentioned previously. If the infection is in a moderately advanced stage, the urine may appear to be cloudy or turbid.

In infants, you will have to watch for more subtle signs: squirming and irritability, more frequent wetting (or infrequent wetting), and an abnormal stream, with fretting and obvious discomfort when urination occurs. If you are suspicious, check the baby's diaper every half hour or so, and you will likely catch the baby in the act of urinating. Then you can evaluate what's going on.

Any urinary tract infection should be seen by a doctor. If a girl has more than two infections in a year, the doctor will probably want to do some detective work to find out why. It could be anything from the way you change diapers to errors in the structure of the urinary system, and it's best to know precisely what the source of the problem is. Urinary tract infections are so unusual in boys that even if your boy has only two episodes over a period of five or six years, your doctor should be consulted.

Urine Testing

To assess whether the kidneys and the rest of the urinary system are working properly, the first thing doctors examine is the urine. This examination has two parts—chemical testing and microscopic examination. A helpful chemical screening can be done at home, using what are known as dipstick reagents. These are strips of plastic that have one to five reagent patches attached. When dipped in a sample of urine, the patches change color, and by comparing the resulting colors with color charts that come with the testing kit, you can easily deter-

mine levels of sugar, ketones, albumin, acidity, bacterial activity, and blood cells in the urine.

These testing kits are available in most drugstores or medical supply stores. Keep in mind, however, that they are not designed to make a definitive diagnosis. If your child has a history of urinary problems, or if you have some reason to suspect a problem may be developing, the dipstick kits can be very useful in helping you judge when to seek professional help. But they are a relatively expensive item, so you would probably only want to have them at your doctor's recommendation or if your child is subject to frequent urinary tract problems. Following are explanations of what a positive result for each of the substances might mean.

SUGAR. Large amounts of sugar in the urine are always abnormal. Diabetes is discussed at length in Chapter 12. If your child has been diagnosed as diabetic and you are specifically monitoring for sugar on a daily basis, your doctor will probably suggest ways to test sugar quantities that are more accurate than urine testing.

KETONES. A positive test for ketones often accompanies a positive sugar test and is most frequently seen in diabetics. Ketones appear in urine when fat is being mobilized and burned by the body. Aside from occurring in diabetes, this occurs in starvation states or at other times when your child may not be eating, because of illness, for example. Children with fevers may mobilize fat reserves because of the increased metabolic demands made on the body. These children will have ketones in the urine without significant amounts of sugar. The ketones will disappear when the fever goes down and the child starts eating normally again.

ALBUMIN (PROTEIN). Substantial albumin in the urine is always abnormal, indicating a problem in the nephrons, the filtering units of the kidneys. A positive test for albumin indicates that protein molecules are being passed through the filtering system along with the water and dissolved salts. This should be called to a doctor's attention. Small amounts may appear after strenuous exercise, and a few normal children regularly have a *trace* of albumin in the urine.

pH (MEASURE OF ACIDITY). A pH of 7 is considered neutral. This is the pH of pure water. Higher numbers indicate an alkaline substance; lower numbers describe acidity. Most body fluids maintain a near neutral pH of just over 7. But gastric juice in the stomach reaches a very acid pH 2; and urine is mildly acid, with a pH 6. Urine may become alkaline for a number of reasons. The child may have been eating slightly alkaline foods. Or there may be a urinary tract infection present. When certain bacteria are present in large enough numbers, they can convert normally acid urine to a higher pH. Then, too, bacteria favor alkaline urine for their growth and are most likely to prosper when urine is somewhat alkaline to begin with. Urine should remain alkaline for more than twenty-four hours, however, before you become concerned.

RED BLOOD CELLS (HEMOGLOBIN). Blood in the urine should never be ignored, even when it appears in minute amounts. Disorders of the bladder often make themselves known with blood in the urine. Sometimes children injure the urethra on riding toys and playground equipment or by poking themselves with sticks or other foreign objects. Kidney trauma—resulting from a blow or fall—can produce bloody urine, or malfunction anywhere in the urinary system can produce blood cells in the urine in greater or lesser amounts. Bleeding can be so heavy that it is obvious as red urine, or it can be so light as to be detectable only with testing. Whatever the case, it calls for a trip to the doctor.

WHITE BLOOD CELLS. If the reagent strip shows an abundance of white blood cell activity, it indicates the presence of an infection somewhere in the urinary system and must be investigated by a doctor.

Bladder and Bowel Control

Control of both bladder and bowel is acquired by most children during the second or third year, but maturing of these controlled functions varies from child to child, and it isn't wise to attempt to toilet train an infant before he is ready for voluntary control. A child must be old enough to understand what a toilet is for and be able to communicate the need to go. Some time before the age of two, most children have achieved enough bladder control to retain urine for two hours or more. At this point, the child should be encouraged to sit on the toilet. First attempts are best made after meals and after naps when the child is likely to void anyway.

Extravagant praise for success and making a small matter of failure are generally considered the best approaches to toilet training. Your baby is as anxious to succeed as you are anxious for success and relief from diapers. Watching father and mother at these chores can furnish a good example of how things are supposed to work, and the child feels grown up doing it on his own. Punishment for accidents that happen beyond an age when you think they shouldn't happen can only have disastrous results. Shaming a child, especially in front of others, will lead to a difficult parent–child relationship that may be hard to repair.

Enuresis

Most, though not all, children can be satisfactorily toilet trained by age three. "Accidents," however, are not unusual through second grade. But continuing lack of bladder control beyond age five should be looked into. The name given to lack of bladder control is enuresis.

There are two types of enuresis—nocturnal, which occurs only at night, and diurnal, which occurs both day and night. Most often, there is no physical cause of enuresis that we know about, but it should be looked into anyway. Urinary tract disorders can lead to frequent urges to urinate, and the increased fluid intake and output of diabetes can lead to lack of control. Children on special medicines and those required to drink large amounts of fluids may also have accidents. If there is a physical explanation, the child must be given maximum support by all concerned. Lavatory privileges in school must be unrestricted.

Treatment of enuresis requires a lot of patience, love, and understanding as it is more painful for the child than for you. Limiting drinks an hour or two before bedtime often helps. Positive reinforcement for each night with a dry bed can be helpful, too. Awarding gold stars or small prizes often brings good results. Certain drugs have been tried with some success for the problem, and devices have been invented that wake a child at the first sign of wetting. These drugs and devices should only be used under the guidance of a physician.

Above all, limit the problem to those who need to know—doctor, teacher, parents. When word gets around among the child's peers, they can make life miserable for him. If the problem persists, psychiatric help may be considered.

Bladder control and control of the anal sphincter come about the same time. Read one of the many good books that tell about training a toddler to toilet or potty. They all have a common theme—it takes praise and patience. There will be successes and failures, and when the child is ready

he will use the toilet regularly. Any effort at coercion, even to the extent of keeping a child on a potty seat longer than he wishes, will only have negative results.

Encopresis

Encopresis is the inability to retain stool or an uncontrolled leakage of liquid stool around an impacted mass of feces in the rectum. Many children with encopresis have encountered premature and coercive attempts at toilet training and have somehow been given the idea that passing feces is a bad thing. Often, these children will have huge and hard bowel movements quite infrequently. After a time, liquid stool begins to leak around the fecal mass in the rectum.

A severe case of constipation in the midst of toilet training may lead to difficulties. If the baby is hurt trying to pass a large, hard stool, she will understandably be reluctant to try again, especially if an anal fissure develops. An anal fissure is a small tear in the anal opening, the result of straining or passing hard feces, and can be quite painful. A few flecks or streaks of bright blood in the stools are the clue. The fissure itself may be hard to see. Treatment of anal fissures is described later in this chapter.

Toddlers, recently toilet trained, will frequently retrogress and experiment with passing their stool in their pants or even somewhere around the house. This is not encopresis and has to be taken in stride as part of your baby's growing up. Less frequently, older children who are generally disturbed will soil themselves as a way to manipulate their parents. Punishment rarely works in such cases, and psychiatric help should be sought.

If you feel you are doing everything right and your child still has difficulties, be sure to involve your physician. There are some unusual physical problems, such as an abnormality of nerves in part of the rectum that could be causing the trouble. If this is the case, you will certainly want to know about it, because there is an operation that usually cures this condition.

Inspecting the Perineal Area

The perineum is the baby's bottom—the area from the coccyx, or tail bone, in back, down between the legs to the pubic bone in front of the genital organs. It's the area you get to know so intimately from changing diapers, and this is the best time to make your inspection. With older children—three and up—bath time is best.

The Anus

All there is to see, of course, is the round, dimpled area with a small opening in the center. The dimpling is caused by the external sphincter muscle, which baby will learn to control with some reliability after age two. You soon get to know what this area looks like when it is normal and well. Any change in appearance signals that something is wrong. Following are some of the more common problems involving the anus.

Inflammation

The skin around the anus is subject to the same irritations as the skin anywhere else. Perineal irritations generally arise from chemical irritation of feces, especially during bouts of diarrhea. The treatment is the same as for diaper rash (see Chapter 2). If the irritation doesn't clear up promptly, consult the doctor.

Anal Fissure

As described earlier, an anal fissure is a small tear in the tissues of the anal opening, usually caused by a large, hard stool passing during constipation. Often it hurts so badly that a child will hold onto the stool, making the constipation worse. Anal fissures appear as cracked lips might, and there may or may not be bleeding. Sit your child in a basin of warm water, with about three teaspoons of salt added, for twenty minutes. Do this three times a day. Dry the anal area gently and apply a small amount of zinc oxide ointment. Keep the child on a diet that will keep the stools soft (see Chapter 4). If your baby is in the process of toilet training, you will want to get the condition cleared up as quickly as possible so that the baby doesn't associate pain with using the potty. If the baby is holding onto the stool and constipation persists, enlist the aid of the doctor in getting rid of the hardened feces.

Anorectal Stenosis

Malformations of the rectum and anus are discovered at birth on rare occasions. The more severe problems are immediately obvious, but sometimes there is simply a narrowing or partial closure of the baby's rectum and anal passageway. This may not become evident until age one or later when you notice that stools are ribbonlike and difficult to pass. This should always be brought to the attention of a physician.

Pinworms

Itching, evidenced by a lot of scratching of the anal area, can be caused by pinworms, called scatworms in some parts of the country. These tiny white worms live in the rectum and emerge to lay eggs on the skin around the anus. It is usually children who bring them home, and they are spread to the rest of the family on towels or even through dust particles in the air that have the microscopic eggs attached to them. A pinworm infestation calls for thorough laundering of clothes and bedclothes, and a blitzkrieg against all dust and dirt in the house that may be mixed with pinworm eggs. Everyone in the family should be treated by a physician.

Discovering pinworms rests with finding pinworm eggs since the worms themselves are usually hiding in the large intestine. It's easy to test for pinworm eggs, but you will need a microscope. Most simple home microscopes or one in a high school lab will do the job.

How to Find Pinworm Eggs

1. Blot around the anal area with the sticky side of a piece of clear cellophane tape. Do this the first thing in the morning before the child gets out of bed. ·

2. Place the tape on a microscope slide, sticky side down.

3. Examine the slide under high magnification. You will see all sorts of debris stuck to the tape, but the pinworm eggs are very distinctive and

unmistakable. They resemble clear chicken eggs, and when you look carefully you can see a pinworm curled up inside.

The External Genitals of Girls

The entire area forward of the anus to the fatty pad of tissue over the pubic bone, with all the structures this area contains, is referred to as the vulva. The vulva is examined by spreading the fleshy outer lips, the labia majora, and checking to see that the area inside is clear, pink, and moist. Check for irritations and discharges. In newborns, you will want to reassure yourself that all the structures are in place pretty much as you see them in the diagram. The inner lips—labia minora—tend to be rather prominent in newborns, but they gradually get smaller, finally becoming almost invisible until puberty when they become larger again. If at any time the inner lips seem to be growing together, or if you suspect the vaginal opening is partly closed, you should call it to the attention of your doctor.

You will encounter few problems in the genital area if you keep the vulva scrupulously clean with gentle washing at every diaper change. Its folds and creases are excellent breeding grounds for

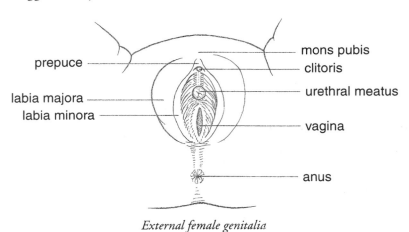

External female genitalia

microscopic organisms; and urine, though initially sterile, quickly deteriorates to become an excellent culture medium for bacteria. Diaper rash, if let go, can invade and irritate the structures of the vulva.

Vaginal Bleeding

Vaginal bleeding can occur in newborn girls anytime between the second and twelfth day of life. The bleeding is usually mild and may last two or three days. This is a normal phenomenon caused by the sudden disappearance of the female hormones that had been previously supplied by the mother, and it is no cause for concern. Other than this, however, vaginal bleeding in young girls should always be investigated by a doctor. Sometimes, in the course of experimenting with her body, a girl will insert something into the vagina. It may cause a cut if it is a sharp object or may result in irritation if left there for any length of time. Unless the object is quite obvious and you are certain it is smooth, have it removed by a physi-

cian. Don't make more of the situation than you have to. It is a normal part of a child's curiosity and urge to explore and experiment.

Vaginal Discharge

Mild discharges are no cause for concern unless they persist for more than a day or two, become heavy, or seem to be mixed with pus or blood. A heavy or persistent discharge can signal vaginal infection and should be treated promptly. Objects inserted into the vagina can cause a discharge that is a mixture of pus and blood. When you visit the doctor because of a vaginal discharge, don't wash the genital area before you go. The doctor will want to take a sample of the discharge for bacterial culture and laboratory examination.

Boys' Genitals

Parents of a first son sometimes find the appearance of their boy's genitals startling: an infant boy's scrotum seems large and pendulous in relation to

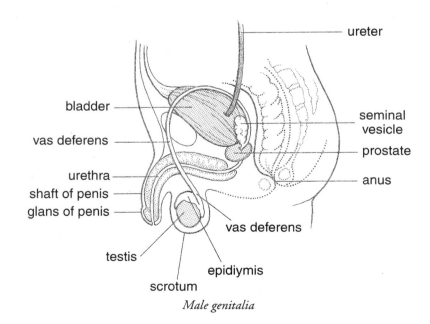

Male genitalia

the rest of him, and for some parents, in this age of widely accepted circumcision, it is their first view of an uncircumcised penis. The prepuce (foreskin) covers most of the head of the penis, or all of it, giving it an unfamiliar appearance for those not used to seeing it that way.

Examination of your boy's genitals doesn't take long, and usually everything is in order; but there are some things to watch for as discussed in the following sections.

The Penis

The urethral opening, the meatus, should be centered in the head of the penis. If the foreskin is covering the opening, you will have to retract it a bit to see. Do this gently, however, because the foreskin in infants is rather tight for the first few months. If you meet resistance, stop; a good jet of urine will tell you that the urethra and its opening are in good working order. If the meatus is not centered, or if the penis seems to have an unusual curved look to it, inform the doctor. If, at any time during childhood, a strong urinary stream narrows, the doctor should be told.

Circumcision

Many parents elect to have a boy circumcised. In recent years, however, some people have questioned the wisdom of circumcision when it isn't required for religious reasons, suggesting that it causes physical and psychological trauma to the child. Others feel that trauma is rare, that the child can be easily comforted and reassured afterward by the mother or father, and that avoidance of future problems with an unnecessary foreskin is well worth having it off in the first days of life rather than later when it is definitely traumatic. Discuss the matter with your doctor before the baby is born so that you don't have to make a snap decision at the last moment.

How to Care for Your Baby Boy's Circumcised Penis

Most circumcisions are simply covered with a gauze dressing impregnated with petroleum jelly. This should be removed forty-eight hours after the circumcision. Then, the area should be gently cleaned with water during diaper changes. Further application of petroleum jelly is unnecessary and soap may be irritating. The following are signs of problems you should watch for.

1. The penis is normally somewhat red after circumcision. If redness increases, or if there is any other change in color—to blue or black— inform the doctor.

2. A few drops of blood is not unusual. Any more bleeding than that should be reported to the doctor.

3. On the second day, you may notice a white fluid oozing from the circumcision site. This is a normal part of the healing process. Copious drainage of fluids or signs of pus are not normal and should be reported to the doctor.

4. The circumcision should be no more than minimally tender by the third day. If soreness persists to the fourth day, inform your doctor.

5. If swelling develops or if you notice the urine stream is becoming weak or dribbling, see your doctor.

6. If the baby begins to act sick and develops a fever, don't delay in seeing the physician.

7. Occasionally a small tag of foreskin tissue is left behind after the circumcision. This is not of immediate concern, but the doctor will want to remove the tag on one of your regular visits.

Boys who have not been circumcised will need some care of the foreskin and may occasionally have problems with it. Infants have tight foreskins, and these should not be forcibly retracted. The danger is that it can become stuck behind the head of the penis; the penis swells and the child can't pass urine. This is an urgent medical situation and requires immediate attention by a physician. Also call the doctor if the foreskin becomes swollen, if there is pus coming from the end of the penis, or if the end of the foreskin is closed, obstructing the urine stream.

Beginning between six and twelve months, the foreskin can be retracted once a week during bathing for gentle cleansing and then returned to its original position. Each time, it needs to be retracted only once. Never force it. Be sure not to leave soapy water under the foreskin as this will cause irritation. Some time between the age of four and five, boys should be taught to do this themselves as a weekly regimen.

If the foreskin becomes mildly inflamed and there is itching or discomfort, you may not be cleaning thoroughly. If the foreskin seems to be stuck, ask the doctor to check it and retract it. Afterward, retract the foreskin three times a day and clean it with mild alcohol or another mild antiseptic solution, rinse, dry, and carefully draw the foreskin forward after each cleaning.

The Scrotum and Testicles

As you can see from the diagram of male genitalia, there are three principle structures in the scrotal sac: the testes, which produce sperm and certain male hormones; the epididymides (singular: epididymis) leading out of the testes, where sperm migrate in adults to mature into their fertile state; and part of the vas deferens, or seminal duct, a long tube that carries sperm to the urethra of the penis.

These structures develop in the abdominal cavity of the fetus and move downward, entering the scrotum shortly before birth. However, about 3 percent of full-term boys are born with one or both of the testicles undescended. Among premature boys, 30 percent have this problem, and the scrotum on "premies" tends to be smooth and shiny, while a full-term baby's scrotum has the more familiar wrinkled, rough appearance with slightly darker pigmentation than adjoining parts of the body. Most undescended testicles will descend between the second and twelfth months of life. If a testicle hasn't descended after a year, your doctor may want to try hormone therapy to bring it down. If this won't work, the doctor will probably recommend that a simple surgical procedure be done before age four or five. At one time, this surgical repair was put off until puberty, but the current trend is toward the much earlier operation.

The testicles are most easily examined in a warm bath since they and the scrotum reflexively draw toward the body in response to a cold touch. The warmth of the water helps keep them descended. Feel for the presence of the testicles, and the spermatic cord, which contains the seminal duct plus nerves, blood vessels, and muscle tissue. You should also feel for anything that shouldn't be in the scrotum.

UNDESCENDED TESTICLE. Feel the scrotal sac gently for two testicles; each is characteristically oval and just over half-an-inch long. Each testicle is suspended by a spermatic cord, so if you find a testicle you will surely find the cord, too. It may take several attempts before you can decide for sure if a testicle is present. If after several attempts, you can't feel one or both, ask your doctor to check on your next visit. There is no urgency or cause for concern about this.

INGUINAL HERNIA. A hernia occurs when some organ or structure in the body moves beyond its normal area into an adjoining part of the body. In an inguinal hernia, part of the intestine moves into the groin area or the scrotum. In the fetus, a retaining wall develops between the abdominal cavity and the groin. If this wall doesn't develop completely, part of the intestine may slip into the groin when baby strains at crying or at other times. Inguinal hernia occurs in about 5 to 10 percent of male babies (it is rare in girls) but may not always present itself in infancy. It may not develop until later in childhood or not until adult life.

An inguinal hernia on one or both sides can be felt as a mass in the groin or in the scrotal sac just above the testicle. Gentle pressure may "reduce" the hernia—that is, the piece of intestine will return to its proper place.

The hernia may appear when baby cries and then reduce itself when he is at rest. Inform the doctor if you discover a hernia. It should be kept under observation to be sure complications don't arise, and at some time in the future, the breach in the abdominal wall will have to be repaired in a simple surgical procedure.

HYDROCELE. A hydrocele also feels like a mass in the testicle, but it is a fluid-filled sac within the scrotum rather than a loop of intestine. Unlike a hernia, a hydrocele cannot be reduced with pressure or manipulation. It just stays in place. You can use a flashlight to distinguish between a hydrocele and a hernia:

- Switch on the flashlight and hold it against the back side of the scrotum.

- If the mass lights up and glows like an orange light bulb, it is most likely a hydrocele. If the light doesn't pass through, the mass is more likely to be a hernia or some other growth.

A hydrocele is not dangerous, but it can be uncomfortable and will have to be corrected. Tell your doctor about it.

TWISTED TESTICLE. Pain in the testicle or groin should always have medical attention. Occasionally one testicle may become twisted within the scrotal sac, inhibiting the flow of blood in the spermatic cord. The scrotum will be extremely tender and there will be moderate to severe pain in the groin above the testicle. It is an urgent situation and requires immediate attention, because with the blood supply cut off, there is danger of losing the testicle. If you can't see your doctor at once, a trip to the emergency room is in order.

CHAPTER 12

WHAT YOU SHOULD KNOW ABOUT YOUR BABY'S ENDOCRINE GLANDS AND HORMONES

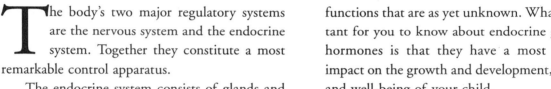

The body's two major regulatory systems are the nervous system and the endocrine system. Together they constitute a most remarkable control apparatus.

The endocrine system consists of glands and specialized groups of cells scattered about the body. These communicate and interact with one another and with other body systems through chemical substances that they secrete directly into the bloodstream. These substances are the hormones. The word *hormone* was created from a Greek word meaning to impel. Essentially, hormones impel cells and organs of the body to act in ways that keep the life systems going—growth, the production of heat and energy, the reproduction processes, and so on.

Most of what we know about endocrine glands and hormones first came to light in the twentieth century, and there are still many mysteries about the endocrine system waiting to be solved. Almost certainly, there are hormones lurking around in the bloodstream waiting to be identified, and there are cells and structures in the body that have endocrine functions that are as yet unknown. What is important for you to know about endocrine glands and hormones is that they have a most important impact on the growth and development, the health and well-being of your child.

Following are the known endocrine glands and some of their main functions:

THE PITUITARY. Located at the base of the brain, it is often called the master gland because it controls or affects the function of other endocrine glands throughout the body. Among other things, it affects growth in children.

THE THYROID. This gland is located at the front of the neck. Its main job is to control the rate at which body cells produce and use energy.

THE PARATHYROIDS. There are four, one at each corner of the thyroid gland. They are important in the control of calcium metabolism which, in turn, affects the function of bone, muscle, and nerve tissues.

THE ADRENALS. There is one atop each kidney. The adrenals have a number of functions, the best known being the shot of energy they stimulate in crisis situations. They also control levels of salt and other important body chemicals.

ISLANDS OF LANGERHANS. These are clusters of cells in the pancreas that produce insulin, necessary to control metabolism of carbohydrates.

THE OVARIES. Located low in the abdominal cavity, the hormones they produce are responsible for the development of female sex characteristics, and they control ovulation and the menstrual cycle.

THE TESTES. Special bodies called Leydig cells in the testicles produce male hormones that are needed for the development of male sex characteristics.

The Pituitary Gland

The pituitary gland is located deep within the head at the base of the brain. It is often called the master gland because some of the hormones it produces stimulate other endocrine glands to secrete their particular hormones. Then, when substances from the other glands reach a high enough level in the body, they stop the pituitary from secreting the stimulating substance. This system of feedback and control characterizes the workings of much of the endocrine system.

The pituitary produces at least six substances and stores others that are produced by cells of the brain. These substances stimulate the thyroid and the adrenal glands, stimulate production of fertile ova and sperm, and help prepare the mammary glands of the breasts to produce milk.

Especially important for children is the pituitary's production of growth hormone, STH (somatotropic hormone). Secretion of too little STH can result in dwarfism, while too much can result in gigantism. Neither condition is common, and both can be caught early by monitoring your child's growth, using the growth charts in Chapter 14. If

any of the following present themselves they should be brought to your doctor's attention.

1. If your child seems to be growing at a rate under the lowest curve of the growth chart

2. If your child seems to be growing at a rate greater than the highest curve of the growth chart

3. If your child falls off the growth line he has been following—that is, if he moves to a higher or lower curve

"My baby seems small," is a common complaint heard by doctors. In most cases, short stature has a very simple explanation in the size of other family members. Nevertheless, measure your baby regularly and record her height and weight on the appropriate charts. If there are any deviations from a regular growth pattern, the doctor should be told about it.

The Thyroid Gland

The thyroid gland is located in the neck, just above the point where the collar bones come together with the breastbone. It is the largest of the endocrine glands and sits astride the trachea (windpipe) with one lobe on either side. The thyroid controls the general rate at which the metabolic mechanisms of the body work. Metabolism is the biochemical processes involved in changing oxygen and nutrients into the energy that all of the body systems need to function. Thyroid hormones also help control the rate at which body tissues and systems grow and develop. So all in all, the thyroid gland has an awesome responsibility, but one that it usually carries off without a hitch. Occasionally, though, a thyroid gland will produce too little or too much of its hormones.

Underactive Thyroid Gland

When a thyroid gland is not producing enough of its hormones, the condition is known as hypothyroidism. (The prefix *hypo-* is generally used to mean under, inner, or lesser: hypodermic needle—a needle used under the skin.) Children with an underactive thyroid will tend to be inactive, sleepy, sluggish, constipated, and have poor muscle tone.

Underactivity of the thyroid gland is most worrisome in the first few months of life. This happens with only a few babies, but it is something to be alert for. A baby that is too good should be suspect—one that sleeps too much, cries minimally, and doesn't seem active and alert when awake.

Hypothyroidism in infants retards development of the nervous system, leading to mental retardation, and it also slows skeletal growth. The resulting condition is known as cretinism. Early treatment, however, started in the first week of life, vastly increases the baby's chance for normal development.

Many states now have newborn screening programs designed to detect hypothyroidism in the first weeks of life. Ask your doctor if your state has such a program. If not, it might be advisable to arrange to have the test done anyway. It is not terribly expensive, and since hypothyroidism causes irreversible damage if undetected and is totally correctable if detected early enough, testing is extremely worthwhile.

Overactive Thyroid Gland

If the thyroid is overactive, the condition is known as hyperthyroidism. (The prefix *hyper-* often means over, more, or too much: hyperactive—overactive, hyperacidic—too much acid.)

Hyperthyroidism is unusual in children under ten and rare in children under six. When it does occur, it is five times as common in girls as in boys. The following are the principal symptoms that hyperthyroidism presents:

- Marked sensitivity to changes in temperature
- Hyperactivity—the child seems unable to sit still
- Marked mood variations
- Weight loss in spite of a voracious appetite
- Tremulous movements
- Sometimes the eyes seem to be bulging, giving a wide-eyed, staring appearance
- Growth (in height) may accelerate
- The skin may be warm, flushed, and moist.

Although hyperactivity is one of the symptoms of hyperthyroidism, all hyperactive children are not victims of overactive thyroids. The more common hyperactivity, which usually first becomes noticeable in school-age children, is another matter altogether. The activity, impulsiveness, and short attention span of some school children is little understood and usually requires a combination of emotional and special educational support as well as attention from a doctor.

Goiter

A goiter is an enlargement of the thyroid gland. It has a number of causes and may occur with an underactive, overactive, or even a normal thyroid. On some very rare occasions a baby may be born with a goiter, in which case precautions must be taken to assure proper breathing since the thyroid gland straddles the windpipe. More often, however, goiter is acquired later in life. Two or more generations ago, the most common cause of goiter was iodine deficiency, occurring mainly in people who did not eat seafood, which contains trace amounts of iodine picked up from the ocean. Today, refrigerated shipments make ocean foods common in all parts of the country, and we now have iodized salt as a way to deal with iodine deficiency in large segments of the population.

A goiter is obvious as a swelling at the base of the neck, in front, where the thyroid gland is located. Since goiter can have various causes (not just iodine deficiency), it should always be seen by a doctor. But considering that goiter is quite rare in children, a swelling in the neck would probably be due to some other cause that needs to be investigated by a doctor.

The Parathyroid Glands

There are four parathyroid glands, located one on each corner of the thyroid. These glands control the metabolism of calcium in the body. Calcium is important not only for bone growth but also for proper functioning of the muscles and nerves. Problems arising in the parathyroids come from either overactivity or underactivity. Fortunately, both hyperparathyroidism and hypoparathyroidism are quite unusual in childhood.

Hypoparathyroidism

An underactive parathyroid (hypo) is somewhat more common than an overactive one. A few children are born without parathyroid glands, and these children develop problems within the first few days of life. Others may have an inherited disorder of parathyroid hormone production, and some will develop hypoparathyroidism for totally unknown reasons.

Symptoms caused by an underactive parathyroid include numbness, cramping, weakness, and twitching of arms, legs, hands, and feet. There may also be diarrhea and sometimes a spasm of the larynx. Children with this condition tend to develop infections of the mouth and fingernails, and teeth don't develop the way they should. These conditions are all closely related to calcium metabolism, which the parathyroid controls.

Occasionally, the first sign of hypoparathyroidism is the development of convulsions. Epilepsy and fever-related seizures are much more common causes of convulsions in children. Still, any child who has a first convulsion should have a serum calcium test to rule out problems with the parathyroid.

Many of the individual symptoms of hypoparathyroidism, in fact, are more commonly produced by other conditions. There are, however, two simple tests you can use if you suspect your child might have this unusual disorder. One tests for the Chvostek sign, and the other for the Trousseau sign, reactions named after the men who first identified them.

How to Test for the Chvostek Sign

1. Find a spot on the face three-quarters of an inch in front of the ear and just below the ridge of the cheekbone.

2. Tap this spot on the face smartly with the tip of the middle finger.

3. If there is a spasm of the facial muscles which produces a grimace, this sign is considered positive.

4. Check on the other side of the face.

How to Test for the Trousseau Sign

You will need your blood pressure cuff to do this test.

1. Place the cuff around the child's upper arm.

2. Bring the pressure halfway between the child's systolic and diastolic pressure. (Review the procedure for taking blood pressure in Chapter 3.)

3. Leave the cuff inflated for about five minutes.

4. If there is a parathyroid problem, the child's hand will go into spasm and he will not be able to control its muscle movement. The wrist bends forward, the thumb is drawn in, and the fingers are held straight but they bend in toward the palm. Deflating the blood pressure cuff allows the spasm to relax.

Babies with hypoparathyroidism tend to be very irritable and twitchy. Occasionally, infants on high phosphorus formulas, such as those made with unmodified cow's milk, will develop symptoms of hypoparathyroidism.

Hyperparathyroidism

An overactive parathyroid is considerably rarer than an underactive one. A child with an overactive parathyroid has poor muscle tone and muscle weakness. There may be general apathy (a symptom common to many childhood illnesses that should always be heeded), vomiting, constipation, and weight loss. High blood pressure often develops, and the rhythm of the heart may become irregular. The child may suffer a broken bone after only a small accident.

The usual cause of this rare condition is a tumor on one of the parathyroid glands. Such a tumor can be removed and the results are usually excellent.

The Adrenal Glands

There are two adrenal glands, each about the size of a baby lima bean in an adult, and one of the pair sits on top of each of the kidneys. The adrenal glands have an outer cortex and an inner medulla. Each part acts separately from the other, secreting its own hormones. The outer cortex produces corticosteroids (cortisone is one of these) and hormones that influence the development of secondary sex characteristics. The inner medulla secretes epinephrine (adrenaline), which provides a quick burst of energy when you are frightened or excited.

The most important type of problem with the adrenals in childhood involves errors in the production of hormones that affect the sex characteristics. This can produce a marked enlargement of the clitoris and other genital abnormalities in girls, and an enlarged penis and early development of pubic and facial hair in boys. Babies with these relatively rare defects will also appear to be ill, and there should be no question about seeking medical advice.

Insulin and Diabetes

The most common endocrine problem of childhood is diabetes. There are two kinds of diabetes: diabetes insipidus, a rare form of the disease caused by pituitary failure, and the more common diabetes mellitus, which is caused by a lack of insulin.

Insulin is produced in specialized cells in the pancreas called islands of Langerhans. The pancreas is a long, thin organ that lies behind the stomach and produces enzymes for digestion. Insulin, however, is a hormone.

Diabetes may start at any time and is occasionally seen in the first year of life, although onset at age three or four is more common. And, of course, it may appear at any time after that.

The word *mellitus* means sweet, and the derivation of the term *diabetes mellitus* comes from the earliest method of diagnosing the disease, actually tasting the sweetness in the urine of diabetics.

Until 1921, diabetes was considered a sentence of death when it appeared in children. It was then that the great Canadian physician Frederick Banting and his medical student assistant Charles Best succeeded in isolating the hormone insulin, enabling diabetics to lead relatively normal and otherwise healthy lives.

The onset of diabetes is gradual and subtle. Sometimes, the first indication a parent has that something is wrong is when the child's blood sugar rises so high that he gradually becomes sleepy and lapses into a coma. It is only in retrospect that parents realize that something has been amiss for several weeks or months.

Signs and Symptoms of Diabetes

- *Thirst,* not an ordinary thirst, but more like the kind you have on a hot day after doing strenuous work. It is easy to overlook, however, since it may simply appear as a child's normal liking for juice or soda.

- *Increased frequency of urination.* You may notice your child going to the bathroom much more than he used to. A child who is considered reliably toilet trained may start wetting again.

- *Increased hunger without weight gain.* There may even be some weight loss.

- *A subtle sense that things are not quite right.* This is a more reliable indicator than you may think. A child may be grouchy, tired, not himself, and complain about feeling "upset."

You can test for high levels of sugar in the urine using a dipstick reagent kit, available in most drugstores. A dipstick is a strip of paper that changes color in reaction to chemical substances in the urine. Instructions come with the kit along with a chart that explains the color changes. The test can be done by simply pressing the stick into a baby's wet diaper, but the diaper should be wet with urine only and not soiled with feces.

The dipstick is only a screening test, however, and should not be considered a sure indicator that the baby does or doesn't have diabetes. A positive result (showing a high level of sugar in the urine) should always be brought to the doctor's attention, and more complete and accurate blood testing will be done.

When a child is diagnosed as diabetic, the doctor will prescribe a regimen of education and health maintenance for both the child and the parent that includes diet, regular blood-sugar testing with home testing equipment, and regular injection of insulin. Insulin must be given every day. No diabetic child can be managed with diet or oral medicines alone.

Blood testing at home and at school is a daily routine, along with injections of insulin to which children quickly become accustomed and can do themselves. Then, regularly scheduled tests by the doctor shows how well a child's diabetes is being controlled over a period of months rather than just during one day. Support from parents and teachers is essential, but the child must learn to do these simple chores himself.

If your child develops diabetes, it is important to guard against treating him as an invalid. You must treat a diabetic child as a normal child who happens to have a special problem, not as a patient who happens to be a child. Excess concern during the childhood years may only result in a rebellious teenager who won't care for himself as he should.

Recent studies show that a properly managed diabetic child practicing good health habits can live as long and as normal a life as anyone else. Summer camps for diabetic children are available in many communities. Diabetic children should be encouraged (not forced) to attend. Getting together with other diabetic children forcefully demonstrates to the child that there are many others like him leading happy and normal lives. The camps also provide valuable education and insight into the everyday problems of living with diabetes.

One young man we know, who was diagnosed as a diabetic at age nine and is now a well-adjusted adult active in camping for diabetic children, told his parents that the best thing they ever did for him was to treat him like a regular kid.

There are many good books available (be sure you use one of recent publication), and information is available from the American Diabetes Association, 1660 Duke Street, P.O. Box 25757, Alexandria, VA 22314, or the Juvenile Diabetes Foundation, 432 Park Avenue, New York, NY 10016.

Sex Hormones

Sex hormones are produced in three places—in the adrenal cortex in both males and females, in the ovaries in girls, and in the testes in boys. Relatively small amounts of sex hormones are found in children, and these come mainly from the adrenal cortex. Improper levels of these hormones can result in certain malformations of sex organs, but this is a rare occurrence.

The presence of estrogens and progesterones in girls, and androgens in boys, increases very slowly until about age eleven. Then there is a marked increase as production from the ovaries and testes begins in earnest. The onset of puberty in children is a fascinating subject, and as your child grows older, make it a point to learn all you can about this remarkable mechanism and its results.

Ovarian tumors occasionally occur in young girls, resulting in advanced skeletal growth, early development of sexual hair, and nipple pigmentation. Menstrual bleeding may also occur. These tumors are generally benign and after surgical removal, recurrence is rare. Treatment should be prompt, however, because advances in bone growth can result in short adult stature. (This is because the faster growing bones will stop growing sooner.)

Testicular tumors in young boys are rare. When they occur, they cause precocious sex development—advanced bone growth, growth of the penis, and development of pubic hair.

What is not unusual, though, is a problem with an undescended testicle, which is discussed in Chapter 11.

CHAPTER 13

HOW CAN I TELL IF MY BABY IS SICK?

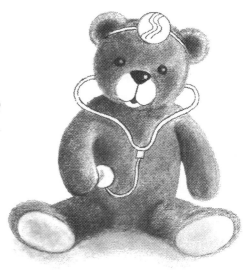

Recognizing illness in a baby or small child can be frustrating. More often than not, it's not at all obvious what the problem is. You can't "see" a fever, an earache, or a slight growth lag, and your infant or toddler certainly can't tell you about it.

Doctors who work with children develop a kind of sixth sense, not unlike a parent's intuition. A pediatrician may say that a baby "looks" (or acts) sick even before the illness has been diagnosed. This instinct alone is reason enough for a doctor to carry out vigorous diagnostic studies.

As a parent, you have an advantage over the doctor because you know how your baby looks, feels, and behaves when she is well. A judgment of illness is always made as a comparison to the healthy state. Your infant may be more active, more fussy, or more precocious than others the same age. Consequently, behavior that may seem normal to a doctor may actually indicate lethargy in this particular baby. In the same way, body temperatures can vary slightly from one child to another. One child's usual body temperature may be a degree lower than average. What might pass for a normal body temperature in most children may actually be a low-grade fever in your child. Knowledge like this is invaluable when examining your baby for the seven cardinal signs of illness: lethargy, fever, inflammation, swelling, lumps, a change in function, and pain.

Lethargy

Lethargy is a telling indicator of illness. The child who is lethargic—or "looking sick," as we say—will sit quietly or perhaps even prefer to stay in bed, when he or she might normally be active. A young infant will lose its usual look of alertness and lie quietly in the crib, looking at nothing in particular. The normal infant activities of moving the limbs and examining the hands and feet may all but cease.

There also may be a subtle change in coloration. The pink-cheeked baby may look sallow, waxy, definitely pale. In darker-skinned babies, you may notice a dusky pallor. In Oriental babies, the faintly yellowish pigmentation of the skin may be heightened during illness.

161

At times, lethargy may be the only sign of illness, and if you believe it represents a substantial change in your baby's or child's usual state, this is good reason to see the doctor.

How to Recognize Lethargy

1. Does your baby or child seem unusually "good," too quiet, reserved, or withdrawn lately?

2. Does she seem to have lost interest in what you're doing or in what her brothers and sisters are up to?

3. Have you noticed an increase in thumbsucking or other self-absorbing activity?

4. If an infant, has the usual crib activity lessened noticeably?

Because lethargic children are less demanding of your attention, their condition may go unnoticed for a while. At some point, however, it suddenly strikes you that the child hasn't "been herself" lately. A "yes" answer to any of the above questions is a clue that something may be wrong.

A stiff neck in a lethargic child is a serious symptom that you should be alert for. If you answered "yes" to any of the above questions, you should check for a stiff neck. A neck so stiff that you cannot bring the chin very close to the chest may be a sign of meningitis, and you should call your doctor immediately.

How to Test for a Stiff Neck

1. Have the child lie flat on his back in bed.

2. You should be able to lift his head so that the chin touches the chest. Your child, of course, must be relatively relaxed and allow you to perform the test.

Fever

Fever is one of the more important signs of illness, and it is the first thing the doctor is likely to ask you about. Measurement of body temperature made with a clinical (mercury) thermometer will be of much greater value to your doctor than a simple statement such as, "My baby feels hot."

RECTAL TEMPERATURE. Body temperature should be taken in the rectum of babies and small children who are unable to hold an oral thermometer in the mouth. The rectal thermometer has a more bulbous-shaped mercury sensor than the oral thermometer.

How to Take the Temperature of an Infant or Small Child

Before you take a rectal temperature, place a small amount of petroleum jelly on the mercury tip of the thermometer; then gently insert it a short way into the rectum, as described below.

1. A good technique to use on infants or uncooperative toddlers is to lay the child, bottom up, on your lap or on a table. Placing the heel of your left hand (or, if you are left-handed, your right hand) on the child's buttocks, spread them apart with your fingers, keeping baby flat so that the knees don't work their way under the body.

2. Gently insert the tip of the thermometer with your free hand, maintaining your hold on the baby's buttocks while the thermometer is in place. If the bulb is one-half to one inch beyond the opening of the rectum, this is quite adequate.

A rectal reading registers quickly. The mercury begins rising almost immediately. When it stops moving, within a minute or so, remove the thermometer.

ORAL TEMPERATURE. By age five, most children can hold an oral thermometer in the mouth. Be certain that the bulb end of the thermometer is kept under the tongue and that the child does not bite down. Instruct the child to breathe through his nose while the thermometer is in place. Three minutes time is generally suffficient for an accurate oral reading.

AXILLARY TEMPERATURE. The axillary temperature refers to the body temperature at the armpit. Place the thermometer as high as possible up under the child's armpit. The arm is then held firmly to the side of the body while the thermometer remains in place for three to four minutes.

SKIN-CONTACT TEMPERATURE INDICATORS. Skin-contact temperature indicators consist of a pliable strip or circle that adheres to the forehead and registers either a digital or a color-coded "read-out." While not as accurate as a mercury thermometer—temperatures are recorded in whole degrees only, and the range is somewhat shorter—you may use them in conjunction with your standard fever thermometer. Take your child's temperature at regular intervals using your mercury thermometer and check with a skin-contact temperature indicator in between times to see if the fever is rising or falling.

EAR THERMOMETERS. These are relatively expensive gadgets you insert in the ear, which take a temperature quickly, provide a digital readout, and even store several readings and the time they were taken. At this time, however, they tend toward gross inaccuracies, even when used in a hospital setting. The presence of ear wax or not getting the instrument firmly seated in the ear can produce a low reading even when there may actually be a raging fever.

Of these methods, the rectal temperature is the most reliable reflection of the actual internal body temperature. Oral temperature is the second most accurate, and axillary comes in third. Normal rectal temperature is approximately one degree higher than normal oral temperature, and axillary temperature is about one degree lower than the oral temperature. When recording temperature, therefore, record not only the reading on the thermometer but the method by which the measurement was made. When reporting a child's body temperature to a physician, do not add or subtract a degree in an attempt to make the temperature comparable to an oral reading. Simply report the numbers and the location.

Once you have taken your child's temperature, the next step is to interpret your findings. Don't be misled by the little arrow pointing at 98.6°F. This supposedly "normal" body temperature is simply a mathematical average that represents many but not all individuals. And body temperature is usually lower first thing in the morning than later in the day. Take your child's temperature several times when she is feeling well, and record this figure in your child's health history for future reference.

Evaluating the Significance of a Fever

THE AGE FACTOR. Fever can vary considerably with the age of a child. A very sick, very young infant may never develop a fever over 100°F. In contrast, a two-year-old may exhibit an extreme fever response and have a body temperature of 104°F with what turns out to be a relatively minor illness. The age of your child is, therefore, an important consideration when evaluating the significance of a fever.

As a general guideline, any fever at all in an infant six months of age and younger should be brought to the attention of a doctor immediately. For a baby six to twelve months of age, call the doctor if the body temperature reaches 100°F. A fever of 101°F in a one-year-old warrants a call to the doctor. By age two, it is safe to wait and see if the fever reaches 102°F and if there is a good response to fever-reducing medication (see below) before calling the doctor.

RESPONSE TO FEVER-REDUCING MEDICA-TION. A relatively reliable method of testing the severity of a fever in children more than a year old is to determine their response to fever-reducing medication—child-size dosage of acetaminophen or ibuprofen. (Aspirin is not recommended as a fever reducer because it has been connected with the potentially deadly Reye's syndrome when given in the presence of a viral disease.)

If a child develops a fever of up to 104°F, administer a dose of nonaspirin, fever-reducing medicine following dosage directions for children on the label. Take the temperature again in an hour or so.

If the child has a relatively mild (usually viral) illness, the temperature is likely to fall approximately one to one-and-a-half degrees, and the child will both feel and act much better. Often children with this kind of illness will lie quietly in bed and look quite ill before you administer the medication, only to be running around the house two hours later. Children with more serious infections, on the other hand, do not show this kind of dramatic recovery. While his temperature may fall in response to the medication, the child will not feel or behave noticeably better.

Monitor fever over the course of an illness. As soon as you realize that the child is feverish, keep a running record of body temperature. Take the temperature three times a day—morning, afternoon, evening. Remember that temperatures taken in the afternoon tend to be higher than morning or evening readings. Be sure to use the same method each time.

If your child's temperature begins to climb after remaining relatively stable or a fever returns after having once subsided, this is an indication that the infection may have spread to a secondary site—such as from the throat to the ears—and you should consult the doctor.

Children with persistent and prolonged fever at any level should be seen by a doctor. Even if the fever is well below 103°F but you think your child is seriously ill or if he is trembling with fever, see your doctor. Any fever at all in an infant younger than six months should be brought to the attention of your pediatrician or family doctor.

Inflammation

Inflammation occurs whenever the blood supply to a specific body area increases beyond what is normally there. Blood circulating through hundreds of thousands of capillaries directly beneath the surface of the skin is what gives the pinkish hue to the bodies of light-skinned people. Capillaries are equally present in dark-skinned people, and they affect skin tone to varying degrees depending on the normal coloring of the skin.

These small capillaries have the capability to enlarge or to contract. When they contract, the skin becomes lighter—obviously pale in whites. Inflammation occurs when the capillaries enlarge and the blood flow through them increases. The area becomes red and often feels hot compared to the rest of the body because more warm blood is being brought to the site of the inflamed area.

Inflammation occurs in response to a noxious (harmful) event. If your baby gets a splinter and it is not removed, the area around the splinter will eventually become swollen and tender, hot and inflamed. Inflammation is one of the body's natural defense mechanisms. In response to the foreign invader—whether it be a splinter, bacteria, or both—the body sends more blood, and particularly more white blood cells, to the area to fight off the invader. Inflammation is therefore a sign that something is wrong and that medical attention is probably necessary.

It is relatively easy to recognize an inflamed hand or foot because you are familiar with its normal coloring. However, unless you have examined the throat, the ear, and other areas of the body when your baby is well, you will find it difficult to recognize the deepening color of inflammation when it occurs.

Recognizing Inflammation

Any part of the body can become inflamed. An inflamed area is red, swollen, and warm to the touch. Patches of inflammation on arms, legs, the back, the abdomen are all obvious, of course. Other areas, like the throat, the ears, and around the excretory openings are less obvious.

IN THE THROAT. You can observe an inflamed throat using a flashlight and tongue blade as explained in Chapter 7. Inflammation in an enclosed area like the throat will make your baby extremely uncomfortable because the associated swelling makes swallowing difficult and painful. Do not take the time to examine your child's throat if he also has a severe, rasping cough and shortness of breath. This combination of symptoms may indicate croup and should be seen by a doctor at once.

IN AN EAR. Inflammation of the outer ear is readily apparent. An inflamed ear lobe will be red, swollen, somewhat shiny, and warm to the touch. You will need an otoscope to detect inflammation in the ear canal. How to inspect the ear using an otoscope is explained in Chapter 5. One good clue to the presence of an inflamed ear is when a fussy baby or child constantly pulls on or pokes at an ear.

Swelling

A swelling is a generalized enlargement of a body part and may vary in consistency from soft to quite firm. Swelling may be associated with inflammation, or it may occur without accompanying heat and redness. Become familiar with your baby's normal pudginess so that you can tell the difference between this and swelling.

Two considerations are important when examining a swelling in your child: the extent of the swelling and its consistency.

Swelling can be either localized or bilateral. Localized swelling is limited to a single body part or area. A bug bite, a blow, a sprain, or a case of poison ivy may result in localized swelling. Look for such a local, or specific, cause whenever swelling is limited to one side of the body—one ear, one eye, one hand, one foot, and so on.

Swelling can also be bilateral—that is, involving both sides of the body, such as both ankles, both feet, or both eyes, or perhaps the whole face. Bilateral swelling is a much more alarming finding than localized swelling because it means the entire body system is involved, not just an isolated part. Severe allergic reactions—to a bee sting, for example, or to a drug—can cause swelling on both sides of the body. Bilateral swelling may indicate the onset of serious illness; therefore, medical attention should be sought promptly.

How to Test for Edema

Bilateral swelling is often caused by an abnormal accumulation of fluid in body tissues, known as edema.

1. To test for swelling caused by edema in the legs, ankles, and feet, press very firmly with one finger against the lower end of the shinbone or against the top of the foot. Maintain firm finger pressure for a slow count of five and then remove your finger.

2. Look closely to see if your finger has left a little dent that can be both seen and felt. If such a dent is apparent, it will gradually smooth out over the next minute or so. Swelling that leaves a dent, or pit, is called pitting edema. Its presence may indicate a serious disorder, which should be investigated by a doctor.

Lumps

Lumps, or masses, as doctors call them, are a fifth sign of illness. Detecting a lump requires considerable familiarity with your baby's body. It's hard to identify a mass in the abdomen, for instance, if you're not sure how your baby's abdomen feels when he is well. It is often possible to feel the edge of the liver in the upper right quadrant of a relaxed infant or child. But unless you have felt this before when your child is well, you may think you've discovered an abnormal mass. In the same way, a bony kneecap felt through a baby's pudgy knee could feel suspiciously like an abnormal bone lump to a worried parent. If, however, you have previously examined your baby's body, you'll be in a much better position to detect a lump that doesn't belong where it is.

Enlarged Lymph Nodes

One of the most common lumps you are apt to find in your child's body is an enlarged lymph node—or lymph gland, as some people call them. The lymph nodes are little nodules of tissue that act as filters. When the body has been invaded by infection, the lymph nodes trap bacteria, viruses, and other debris. As a node accumulates more and more material, it enlarges and you can feel it readily. Enlarged lymph nodes, therefore, are a sure sign that your baby is fighting off an infection of some kind.

Clusters of lymph nodes are located on either side of your baby's neck, under both armpits, and on both sides in the groin area. There are also a few lymph nodes in the area around the elbows and behind the knees. Different clusters drain different parts of the body. Knowing which nodes filter which areas can help you to identify the probable source of an infection.

How to Detect Enlarged Lymph Nodes

Enlarged lymph nodes can vary in size and may feel small, like a piece of buckshot, or larger, like a small almond. They feel firm and hard.

1. With your fingers together, use your fingertips to feel for lymph nodes in the neck at about the jawline and just below.

2. Next feel in the groin where the legs meet the body.

3. Lastly feel your child's armpits.

Lymph nodes under your child's jaw commonly swell as a reaction to a toothache, sores in the mouth, or a viral respiratory infection, such as flu. Swollen nodes behind the ears suggest an ear infection, or perhaps a sore or tick in the scalp. Enlarged nodes in front of the ears point to some problem in the area of the face and eyes. Similarly, an infected toe may cause nodes to enlarge behind the knee or in the groin on that side. If a child has a cut or scrape on one arm, it would not be at all surprising if the lymph nodes in the armpit on that side became temporarily swollen.

A single swollen lymph node or a few enlarged nodes in one localized area most likely indicate a cut or minor infection and are usually not particularly important. Multiple swollen lymph nodes, however, enlarged nodes on both sides of the body, or a single large, painless node that lasts longer than a day or two may indicate a serious problem.

Swollen, tender lymph nodes accompanied by red streaks up an arm or leg indicate serious widespread infection (commonly called blood poisoning) and should be treated as a medical emergency.

The lymph nodes seem to enlarge much more readily in some children than in others. In some, a few lymph nodes on both sides of the neck will pop out every time the child gets a cold and will go away again when the cold is resolved. In others, it may be very difficult to feel the lymph nodes even with a severe cold. Examining your child regularly will help you determine which category she falls into.

Abdominal Masses

There are many causes for abdominal masses, some very serious and others relatively harmless. If your baby or child is crying, curled up and holding her abdomen, look for a mass by palpating, or feeling, the abdomen. Feel each quadrant systematically

and gently, then palpate somewhat more deeply. It is sometimes possible, as we have noted before, to feel the edge of the liver in the right upper quadrant. In the lower left quadrant, a hardish, elongated mass may be compacted feces, related to constipation. If you feel such a mass in this area, see if you can relate it to a recent absence of adequate bowel movements. Abdominal masses vary considerably in size. Something as small as an olive can be very significant, particularly in a young infant. Any abdominal mass in a child who appears to be ill should be brought to a doctor's attention.

Lumps on Bones and in Soft Tissues

Lumps occasionally grow on the bones. These bone masses are most likely to appear near the ends of the long bones—above and below large joints—and feel like hard, immovable bony knots beneath the skin. Compare the opposite member of the body when feeling for bone lumps—both knees, hips, ankles, wrists, arms. Abnormal bone lumps almost never appear in the same location on both sides of the body at the same time. If you find such a lump in your child, consult your doctor promptly.

Both small and large lumps can also appear in soft tissue—under the skin or in a muscle—anywhere on the surface of the body. If these quickly develop to the size of an almond or larger, they may represent an abcess, which should be drained. There are numerous other causes for surface lumps, and medical attention is generally required to get rid of them.

Change in Function

Each of the body systems has its own function to perform. When we are well, we are barely conscious of these functions. The slightest change in the performance of a body system, however, can cause considerable discomfort and is a sure sign that your baby or child is ill.

Diarrhea, constipation, vomiting, a greatly increased or decreased urine output, abnormal breathing sounds, unusually rapid pulse even when resting are all signs that something is wrong. Normal spitting up, on the other hand, is not a change of function, of course. By using a little calm judgment, you can soon learn to distinguish between repeated or persistent stomach upset, which may include vomiting and diarrhea, and an occasional throwing up or transitory "loose bowels," such as you might experience yourself without serious ill effects.

A serious change in the function of the digestive system, however, can result in dehydration as described in Chapter 4. Babies and young children have limited fluid reserves, and with severe diarrhea, these are quickly used up. You should be alert for dehydration when your baby has a digestive complaint or a continuing fever.

Recognizing Dehydration— the Pinch Test

Watch for drying of the lips, tongue, and membranes inside the mouth, which is one of the earliest signs of dehydration. Gently pinch your baby's skin between your thumb and forefinger. Normal skin is elastic and will snap back almost instantly. In a dehydrated baby, however, the skin over the arm and particularly the abdomen develops a doughy consistency; when you pinch it, it will stay heaped up almost like putty for a few seconds. Decreased urinary output and sunken fontanels are other signs of dehydration.

If you suspect your baby is dehydrated, treat this condition as a medical emergency and consult a doctor at once.

Good Babies and Fussy Babies

Finally, an exceptionally good baby or an exceptionally fussy baby may both be cause for concern. Some babies are squally, active, and difficult to take care of, whereas other babies are pleasant, generally quiet, and rarely cry. Both of these are normal. But a baby who is constantly fussing and crying and who can somehow never be made happy for any length of time may have a problem, and most parents will not hesitate to bring this to the doctor's attention. The baby who is "too good," on the other hand, sometimes escapes medical attention because the parents do not perceive anything to be wrong. If your baby sleeps more than you think he should, cries less, and spends most of the time simply staring at the ceiling or gazing blankly into space, an alarm should go off in your head. These "silent symptoms" are another kind of change in function and should be taken as seriously as the squawky kind.

Pain

Of all the signs of illness, pain is the most dramatic. Yet even when its presence is unmistakable, it can be difficult to pin down, especially in babies and small children. Unlike a fever that can be measured or an injury that can be examined, pain is purely subjective—only the person who is in pain knows exactly how it feels. As adults, we have learned to describe pain using such terms as sharp, dull, intense, throbbing, and so on. Children do not have a full set of adult experiences with which to compare any one pain. To them, pain simply "hurts." Babies, of course, cannot even tell you that much.

Finding out where it hurts can be a real challenge for parents. Children tend to localize pain poorly because they may not have the vocabulary to distinguish between an elbow and a knee or a chest and a tummy. Or they can keep repeating "It hurts" without being able to tell you what "it" is. It's worth the effort, however. Tracing your baby's pain to a particular part of the body can help you decide whether or not to call the doctor and what to tell the doctor if you do call.

Checking for Obvious Hurts

Before subjecting a crying baby or toddler to a lengthy examination, make a brief inspection of the body to see if there is an obvious problem. A stone in the shoe, a sliver in a hand or foot, a black-and-blue mark, an insect bite, and so on are all common hurts that might be troubling your child.

Is the baby hungry? Babies don't always get hungry on schedule. See if an extra feeding will help.

Examine the extremities. Gently, but firmly, feel along the length of each arm and leg and carefully move each joint. A child will noticeably wince, cry out, and withdraw the limb from your grasp if you find a sore spot.

Finally, examine the head, neck, and chest. Look for tender areas by pressing gently with the flats of your fingers.

Some children react to minor injuries stoically, with little or no fuss. Others have a much lower threshold for pain. In evaluating the severity of pain, therefore, past experience with a particular child is extremely important.

The presence of continuing or persistent pain anywhere is good reason to seek medical help. Obviously, small children fall, get bumps or bruises, and eat green apples, all of which cause some degree of passing pain. Pain from a bump should go away rather quickly. Stomach upset can last a few hours. Any pain that persists beyond a few hours, that intensifies, or is accompanied by other symptoms should be brought to the attention of a doctor.

Abdominal Pain and Upset

Abdominal pain is probably the most frustrating kind of pain for a parent to deal with. It is the most common ailment of infants and young children, yet it is one of the most difficult symptoms to fathom. A pain in the abdomen can be caused by constipation, a flu bug, colic, a bowel obstruction, a urinary tract infection, or even stress, to name just a few possibilities. Even doctors do some head scratching when their own children complain of a tummy ache.

The problem is in distinguishing between something transient and relatively minor, and something that should be seen by a doctor. Abdominal pain alone is hard to diagnose. Considered in combination with other symptoms or as part of a recurrent pattern, however, it is often possible to determine what the problem is.

In an infant under six months of age, recurring abdominal pain very often turns out to be colic. Colic is the name given to a pattern of recurring episodes of abdominal pains in a very young baby. It is easy to recognize and hard to ignore. Fortunately, colic is temporary and harmless. Three factors help you diagnose the sharp abdominal pains of colic: the age of the baby, the timing of the discomfort, and the characteristic "colic pose."

How to Recognize Colic

1. *Age.* Colic afflicts the very young infant. It commonly develops around the first two to four weeks of age and may persist right through the third month. Colic rarely lasts beyond this period—hence its name, "three-month colic."

2. *Timing.* Colic pains typically strike after a late afternoon or evening feeding. The crying usually begins within a half-hour of feeding and continues for as long as four hours, until the next feeding. Colic pains may recur day after day, with striking regularity.

3. *The colic pose.* A baby suffering from the sharp abdominal pains of colic assumes a characteristic pose with the legs drawn up to the abdomen and the fists clenched. The abdomen is somewhat distended with gas, and the hands and feet may feel cold and moist to the touch.

Despite recurrent episodes of obvious pain, colicky babies thrive and continue to gain weight, and most doctors agree that colic is harder on the parents than on the baby.

If you have ruled out colic as a reason for abdominal pain, look for other symptoms to help you decide how serious the problem is. Vomiting, diarrhea, and fever are all symptoms that may accompany abdominal pains. Abdominal distress accompanied by a noticeable decrease in bowel movements may mean constipation.

A combination of abdominal pain, distended abdomen, and projectile vomiting, in which the vomitus is expelled with considerable force from the mouth, suggests a bowel obstruction and should be treated as a medical emergency.

Abdominal pain accompanied by vomiting and diarrhea typically occur with intestinal flu; dehydration is a major cause of concern here, especially in young babies. Fever may accompany any of these problems, indicating that the body is fighting off an infection of some kind. Finally, a complaint of a tummy ache that is not accompanied by a change in bowel habits, vomiting, diarrhea, or fever, and that does not interfere with TV watching or story time is probably of no great consequence.

Just as in any other life situation, judgments about illness and what you do about it are based on combinations of circumstances and on experiences you have had in the past. For example, you learn quickly about spitting up after your baby's feeding, and it doesn't alarm you. Repeated or frequent vomiting, your own good sense tells you, should be investigated by a doctor. A baby who is fussy about one feeding is not necessarily a sick baby, but a baby who keeps refusing food and has other symptoms—such as fever, lethargy, persistent watery diarrhea—needs medical attention.

The seven signs of illness pertain to illnesses with rapid onsets—anything from a few hours to a day or two. Some illnesses develop very gradually, however. In these cases, the more dramatic danger signs will generally be absent. Fever and pain will usually not play a prominent role. Slow-onset illness is marked by a slowing or cessation of the growth rate and, perhaps, weight loss. This is why it is important to plot your child's growth on the standard growth charts provided in Chapter 14, "Tracking and Testing Your Child's Growth and Development."

Ultimately, the surest indicator of a baby's well-being is a parent's own intuition. No one knows a baby better than her parents, and no one is in a better position to notice the slight changes in behavior that can be every bit as revealing as the more conventional symptoms of illness. Just as you can tell with a look whether or not your spouse is out of sorts some days, you can also "read" your baby's health in an educated glance. Unscientific as it may be, this kind of diagnosis tends to be uncannily accurate and should never be ignored.

Fortunately, well babies are the rule and sick babies are the exception. Even as a first-time parent with no experience and a lot to learn, you won't make many mistakes, and you will probably judge on the side of caution rather than on the side of recklessness with your baby's well-being. If you are alarmed and you don't trust your judgment when faced with a certain combination of circumstances, never hesitate to consult your doctor without embarrassment. Educating parents is as important a part of a doctor's job as treating the occasional illness that may arise. If your fears are groundless, the doctor should explain why, and you will have learned a valuable lesson for next time.

CHAPTER 14

TRACKING AND TESTING YOUR CHILD'S GROWTH AND DEVELOPMENT

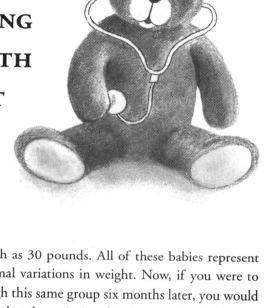

Some parents expect all children of the same age to be at about the same level of growth and development. But it doesn't happen that way. One eighteen-month-old may be 30 inches in length, while another measures a full 34 inches. Both are normal, and so is anything in between. The same goes for weight, head circumference, and the developmental skills, such as walking and talking. In fact, compare one child with another and you are likely to come up with more differences than similarities.

However, though you cannot compare your child with one other, you can compare your child with a thousand others or ten thousand others, and come up with a reliable assessment of his growth and development. On average, babies of the same age tend to fall within certain ranges of development, and they continue to grow and develop at predictable rates.

If, for instance, you were to weigh a thousand eighteen-month-old boys, you would find that the majority of them weigh about 25 pounds. A few would weigh as little as 21, and another few, as much as 30 pounds. All of these babies represent normal variations in weight. Now, if you were to weigh this same group six months later, you would find that the majority, this time, weighed about 28 pounds, with the same few lightweights weighing in at about 23, and the bigger ones from last time now tipping the scales at about 33. Moreover, you'd find that each baby had maintained his relative position within the range of normal variations. In the long run, the small babies will always be smaller than average, and the large ones, larger than average.

What you want to know and what your doctor wants to know is that your baby's rate of growth is proceeding as expected. And you surely want to know if it slows, accelerates, or stops. The only way to know if this is happening (and in time to do something about it) is to measure your baby regularly and compare his progress with what is expected of him.

The tools you use to compare his progress are the same ones pediatricians rely on—the growth charts compiled by the National Center for Health

173

Statistics (NCHS). Fourteen of these charts are included in this chapter, with instructions on how to duplicate the precise measurements taken by your doctor.

Plotting Your Child's Growth Curves

Each NCHS growth chart deals with only one kind of measurement—head circumference, weight, or height—as it relates to the child's age. (The only exception is the stature–weight chart, which you use to determine whether your child's weight is appropriate for her height.)

The information is presented in graph form. There's one scale across the bottom (usually for age), and a second scale up the side for weight, length, or whatever is being measured. The graph itself has five curving lines. These are labeled 5th, 25th, 50th, 75th, and 95th, indicating the part or percentile of the population in which your child is tracking.

The middle line—the 50th percentile—represents the average or median course of growth found in a large sampling of children. Many children, as they grow, grow at the rate indicated by this middle line. The bottom line, or 5th percentile, shows the rate of growth that will be followed by the smallest babies—roughly 5 out of every 100. The top line, or 95th percentile, shows the course that will be followed by the largest babies—again, about 5 out of every 100. All of these growth patterns are normal. Children can even fall slightly outside of these top and bottom lines and still be normal. When you measure your child's growth regularly and plot the results on the appropriate graphs, you will soon see a growth pattern emerging that is roughly parallel to one of the percentile curves.

By the time your child is a few months old, and certainly by one year of age, she should have established herself on or parallel to one of the five growth curves. By the time a child is one year old, if you have made measurements every month or two, you should see that she is continuing to grow regularly along this line.

Interpreting Your Child's Growth Line

More important than knowing just where within this family of lines your child falls is watching to see if he continues to grow along his established line. For example, if your child is growing in length along the 50th percentile curve and then, at age one year, slows his growth so that, at fourteen months, he is on the 25th percentile line, you should be concerned. Once a child establishes his "channel," it should be expected that he will follow this same course over the full span of childhood development. A change in growth curve is always an important reason to check with your doctor.

Continued normal growth is a critical consideration. It is also one area that parents can evaluate better than doctors. Most doctors (but not all) weigh and measure their young patients each time they see them. At the beginning, this may be once a month. Inevitably, though, these visits fall off, until your child sees the doctor only once each year or when she's ill. Parents, on the other hand, can measure their baby regularly and plot these measurements on the appropriate growth charts. They can confirm, at the earliest possible time, whether or not their baby's growth rate is progressing normally.

The three most important measurements are head circumference, length (or height), and weight. Chest and abdominal circumference are often measured as well, but are of lesser importance in following the growth of the baby after she comes home from the hospital.

Measuring Your Baby's Head Circumference

An infant's head grows at a fairly rapid rate, especially in the first six months of life, which is the critical period for detecting abnormalities in this area. You should measure your baby's head circumference every month for the first year, and you may wish to continue to take this measurement every three months to six months thereafter until your baby is three years old.

How to Measure Head Circumference

1. Using an ordinary tape measure, place it around the baby's head at the point of maximum circumference. This is usually just above the brow, right above the ears, and around the back of the head. Make several measurements until you are convinced you have measured the largest circumference.

2. Write down the measurement you have just taken. Now go to the appropriate chart. The first chart is for girls, the second, for boys. Find your baby's age along the age scale.

3. Next, find your baby's head circumference on the head circumference scale. Follow the head circumference line horizontally until it intersects the vertical line representing your baby's age. Make a small *X* at this point.

4. Note which percentile line your marks lie closest to. Plot a new *X* on the chart every month.

5. Then, draw a line connecting the *X*s.

As the months go by, the line should follow one of the lines on the chart or run parallel to one of the lines. If the line you make begins to cross lines into another percentile, call this to your doctor's attention. Tracking head circumference on a regular basis can help you detect a relatively uncommon but potentially life-threatening condition called hydrocephalus.

This is an abnormal accumulation of fluid within the skull and shows itself as an enlargement of the head. If you suspect your baby's head circumference is abnormally large, or if it seems to be increasing faster than the chart indicates it should, consult your doctor at once.

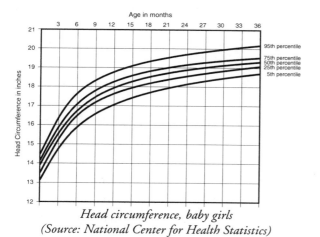

Head circumference, baby girls
(Source: National Center for Health Statistics)

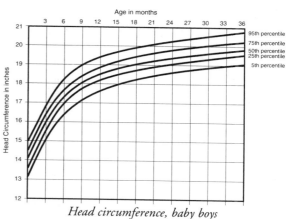

Head circumference, baby boys
(Source: National Center for Health Statistics)

Tracking Your Baby's Length

Determining a baby's length is probably the trickiest measurement to record accurately. Babies tend to squirm, and they prefer to lie with their legs somewhat bent at both the hips and the knees rather than absolutely straight out. So, be sure that the baby is stretched out as straight as possible at the time the measurement is taken.

How to Measure Length

1. Place the baby on his back with the soles of his feet flat against a firm surface, such as the footboard of the crib.

2. Straighten the baby's legs and body as much as possible and then stand a book or some other straight object upright so that the flat surface just touches the top of the baby's head.

3. Now, measure the distance between the footboard and the book with a yardstick or a tape measure stretched tightly.

4. For greatest accuracy, repeat the entire process three times and average your results.

Take new measurements every three months, and plot your baby's increasing length on the appropriate chart. Again, look for a pattern that parallels one of the percentile lines and, once a line is established, be alert for any falling off from this established rate of growth.

Measuring Your Baby's Stature

Between ages two and two-and-a-half, your child should be able to stand upright with feet together and should be measured in this position. Doctors refer to this measurement as stature, which can be

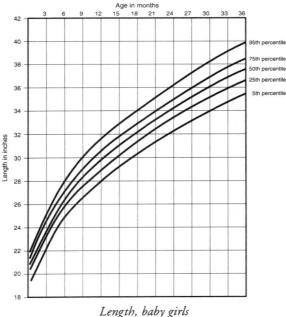

Length, baby girls
(Source: National Center for Health Statistics)

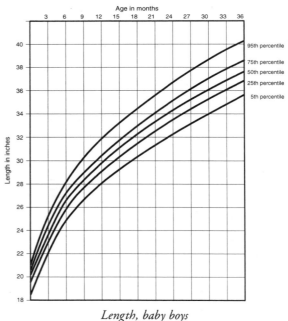

Length, baby boys
(Source: National Center for Health Statistics)

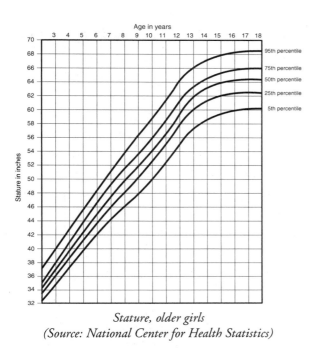

Stature, older girls
(Source: National Center for Health Statistics)

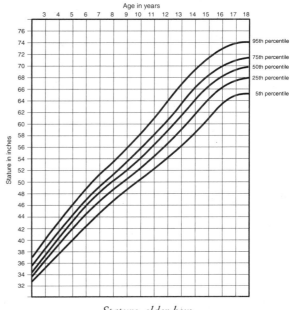

Stature, older boys
(Source: National Center for Health Statistics)

thought of simply as length standing up, or what most of us call height.

How to Measure Stature

1. Stand your child, barefoot, against a wall or door frame.

2. Place a ruler on top of her head and, holding it absolutely horizontal, touch it to the wall or door frame behind her. Make a small mark on the wall where the ruler touches.

3. Measure from the floor to your mark.

Many parents make these marks using a permanent marker such as a felt-tip pen, and they write the date next to the mark. Eventually, your wall will display a growth record for each child. Older children find it entertaining to look back on their own growth records kept this way.

Included here are the NCHS stature charts to use in plotting stature from ages two through eighteen. Make a new entry on the chart at least twice a year. Be consistent. It is just as important for older children to follow a regular growth curve as it is for younger ones.

Measuring Your Baby's Weight

Weight gain—or lack of weight gain—is a telling indicator of your baby's health. Weigh your baby at least every three months, and track weight gains on the appropriate NCHS growth chart.

A reminder: every baby loses about 10 percent of his birth weight during the first few days of life. A six-pound baby, for example, may lose as much as ten ounces, a nine-pound baby almost a pound. So what looks like a setback is, in fact, perfectly normal. From the time your baby is ten days

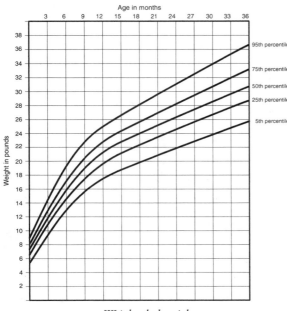

Weight, baby girls
(Source: National Center for Health Statistics)

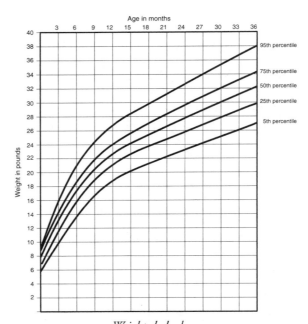

Weight, baby boys
(Source: National Center for Health Statistics)

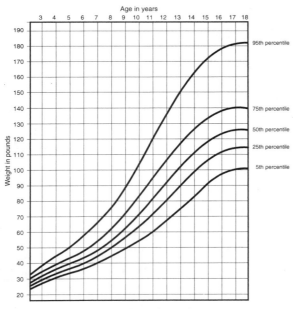

Weight, older girls
(Source: National Center for Health Statistics)

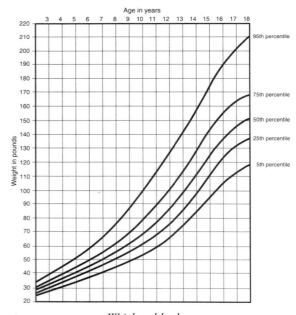

Weight, older boys
(Source: National Center for Health Statistics)

old, however, she should start exhibiting steady weight gains.

How to Measure Weight

1. *Using a bathroom scale.* To weigh a child up to about age two on an ordinary bathroom scale, first weigh yourself. Record that weight.

2. Next weigh yourself holding the child and record the combined weight of yourself and the baby. You can then determine the baby's weight by subtracting your weight from the combined weight. This method is only accurate to the nearest pound or so. *Note:* It is very important to use the same bathroom scale for all measurements; it is common for such scales to vary from one to another by as much as three pounds.

3. *Using a small table scale.* A small table scale, or a baby scale with a basket, provides a more accurate record of an infant's weight because it shows fractional variations in weight. These show up at tag (or yard) sales fairly often. Use a five-pound bag of sugar to check accuracy.

4. If you use an ordinary table scale, you must first weigh a suitable lightweight basket or board on which the infant can lie; then subtract the weight of this device from the total.

A note of caution: use extreme care in weighing an infant on a table scale. Because of the small surface of the weighing platform, the basket or board holding the baby can easily tip off if the baby wiggles or rolls. For this reason, the scale should always be placed on the floor, preferably on a soft carpet. It should never be used in its usual location on the kitchen counter. Moreover, keep your hands close to the baby while he is being weighed.

Try to make weight measurements under the same circumstances each time. For example, after a bowel movement and before a feeding are good times to weigh your baby, just as you would weigh yourself when following a diet or exercise regimen.

As a rule of thumb, you can expect your baby to gain about one ounce each day during the early months of life. Birth weight has generally doubled by the fourth or fifth month, tripled by the end of the first year, and quadrupled by the end of the second year. On average, children between ages two and nine gain about five pounds a year.

By tracking your baby's weight on the growth charts, you should see at a glance whether she is adding the weight she should. The first two charts follow weight gains from birth through age three (one for girls and another for boys). The last two charts are for tracking weight through age eighteen.

Checking Weight Versus Length

By itself, an individual's weight is not a particularly revealing figure. Is 130 pounds a desirable weight for a young woman? It depends, of course, on whether she's 5'7" or 5'0". A child's weight should be proportional to height, too. For this reason, the NCHS has devised a set of growth charts comparing length with weight.

For example, a five-year-old boy who weighs 32 pounds is tracking on a low percentile on the age-weight curve, between the 5th and 10th percentiles. You might say he's light for his age. But if he stands just 3'5" tall, his weight is about proportionate to his height. He is on a low

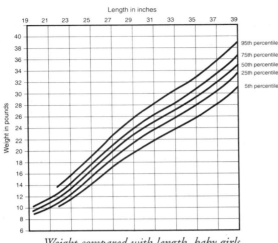

Weight compared with length, baby girls
(Source: National Center for Health Statistics)

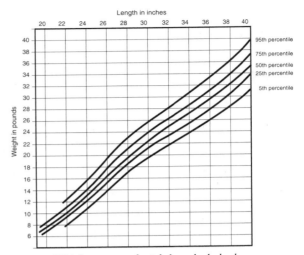

Weight compared with length, baby boys
(Source: National Center for Health Statistics)

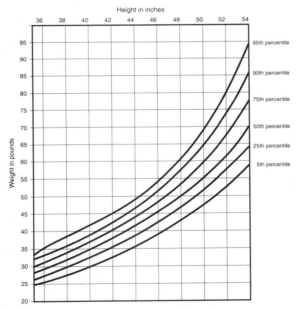

Weight compared with height, girls ages three to ten years
(Source: National Center for Health Statistics)

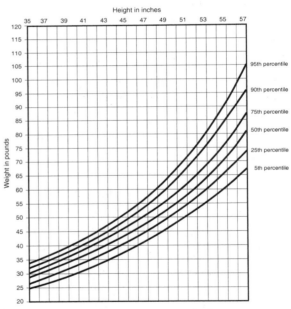

Weight compared with height, boys ages three to ten years
(Source: National Center for Health Statistics)

percentile curve here as well. However, if this same 3'5" boy weighs 50 pounds, his weight is not in proportion to his height. His height is tracking on

a low percentile curve, while his weight is tracking beyond the 95th percentile. He is quite overweight.

So on the weight–length charts, there are two things to watch for:

1. Is your child tracking on about the same percentile line as on the age–weight and age–height charts?

2. Is your child following one curve pretty consistently—that is, no crossovers to a new curve that may indicate a sudden change in the growth pattern?

If the answer to either of these questions is "no," discuss your observations with your doctor.

What Size Will My Baby Be?

It's hardly a matter of medical importance, but parents who take advantage of end-of-season sales want to know, "How big will my baby be next year?" You can use the same NCHS charts you use to plot your baby's growth to project how much taller and how much heavier she will probably be three months, six months, or a year or more from now.

Once your child has established her own growth line on the NCHS charts, you can make an educated guess at future growth using the percentile curve she most closely follows. If, for example, your one-year-old girl weighs 23 pounds and has been growing along the 50th percentile, you can continue along this curve and "guesstimate" that at eighteen months she'll weigh about 24 pounds, at age two, about 27 pounds, and so on. Similar calculations can be used to project length and stature.

All bets are off, however, when a child approaches puberty. Some teenagers who were big children stop growing early, and some small youngsters keep on growing and end up tall. Final adult stature is hard to predict.

Developmental Milestones

As your baby grows, his brain and nervous system are developing, too. This development is responsible for the increasing complexity of your baby's skills and movements. Flailing arms and legs gradually come under control, coos and babblings turn into meaningful sounds. Before long, the baby who at birth was little more than an appealing bundle of reflexes has developed many skills and accomplishments.

Doctors refer to new achievements as developmental milestones. These milestones include things such as head control, grasping objects, and making the sounds that later become speech.

There are literally dozens of developmental milestones, classified as gross motor skills, fine motor skills, language development, and social development. Some milestones are more significant than others, and such key milestones—as we will call them—are landmarks of your baby's progress. Each of these landmarks is proof that your baby has mastered a rather complex sequence of skills. If your baby achieves the four key milestones designated in each of the four developmental areas—gross motor, fine motor, language, and social—you may rest assured that he is doing fine. (The key milestones are described a little later in this chapter.)

Like the growth statistics presented earlier, there's considerable variation within the normal range of skills development. Some babies walk long before others, some much later. It depends on the individual rate of maturation of the nervous system. Sooner or later is rarely a cause for concern and has little bearing on a child's abilities later in life. Marked delays are, of course, a matter of concern. If there is a milestone that is much longer coming than indicated as an outer limit, this situation should be discussed with your doctor.

Make a Photographic Record

A good way to record developmental milestones is with a still or video camera or camcorder. Photographing a child standing alone, without support, is a sure way of demonstrating that the child has, indeed, attained a particular milestone. If photographs are taken with the specific aim of recording developmental milestones, they will form a graphic and interesting review of your baby's achievements. Be sure the pictures are dated.

You might also photograph your baby regularly in front of the same background—the living-room fireplace, for example—to highlight your baby's growth in relation to an object that remains the same.

Gross Motor Milestones

The term *gross motor movements* refers to movements made by the large muscles—the ones controlling the arms and legs, the head, and the torso. The gross motor milestones include dramatic achievements such as crawling, standing, and walking. These are momentous events and are hard to miss.

Babies possess certain motor abilities at birth, but most of these are little more than reflexes. For example, if you hold your baby under his arms in an upright position and touch his feet to the floor or mattress while moving him forward, he will make walking movements. This is a reflex action and does not indicate the development of walking ability. Similarly, if the baby is lying on his back and you make a loud noise or slap your hand down on the mattress, he will make a grasping motion with both arms. This, again, is a reflex action and does not suggest precocious motor development.

The key gross motor milestones you should watch for are these: head control, rolling over, sitting without support, and walking.

HEAD CONTROL, TWO TO FOUR MONTHS. The ability to control head movements is among baby's first motor milestones. By age three months, the average baby will be able to hold his head upright when he is held in a sitting position. A few infants will be able to do this at about five weeks of age, and some normal babies will not be able to hold their heads steady until they are four months old.

HEAD CONTROL, THREE TO FIVE MONTHS. A developmental test popular with pediatricians is checking the ability of a baby to be pulled by the arms to a sitting position without having the head lag backward. The average baby develops this ability at about seventeen weeks, a few as early as thirteen weeks, and some not until twenty weeks.

ROLLING OVER FROM FRONT TO BACK, THREE TO SIX MONTHS. This is a very important milestone because parents often turn away from babies when they are lying on the bed or on the diaper-changing table, assuming that they will not be able to move away. This should never be done. It is truly remarkable how unexpectedly babies acquire new skills. Unfortunately, they seem to choose the worst possible moment to perform their new trick. Expect the unexpected and keep your eye and at least one hand on your baby during changing times.

ROLLING OVER FROM BACK TO FRONT, FOUR TO SEVEN MONTHS. It takes longer for a baby to learn to roll over from back to front. This may not occur until six or seven months.

SITTING WITHOUT SUPPORT, SEVEN TO TEN MONTHS. Sitting without support signifies considerable muscular development, coordination, and balance. The majority of six- or seven-month-old babies are able to sit with their backs supported or with hand support. Some can do this earlier. By the age of eight to ten months, your baby should be able to sit without support, steadily, and with his back straight.

WALKING, TEN TO SIXTEEN MONTHS. Walking alone is the milestone many parents consider the most important of all. On the average, this occurs at about one year. Some babies will begin walking shortly after they are eleven months old, and most are walking by fourteen months. A few perfectly normal babies will not walk until they are sixteen months old.

Fine Motor Milestones

The term *fine motor movements* refers to the precise movements made by the smallest muscles. Fine motor movements are not nearly so dramatic to observe as gross motor movements, but, in the long run, it is the fine motor movements that enrich your child's life. Writing, drawing, sewing, assembling a model, and playing a musical instrument all require fine motor movements. But then, so do picking up cookies, dumping things out of cans, pulling things out of drawers, and turning on faucets. Most children prove to be adept at all of these things.

Again, some fine motor skills are more significant than others. Four key milestones in this area are the whole-hand grasp, the pincer grasp, the two-block tower, and scribbling ability.

THE WHOLE-HAND GRASP, TWO TO FOUR MONTHS. A newborn baby will clench your finger in his fist when you touch it to the palm of his hand. This is purely a reflex action. Within a few months, however, your baby should display the first signs of fine motor development by closing his hand around an object, such as a rattle, and holding it for a short time before it falls out of his grasp. Some babies develop this ability by two-and-a-half months; a few do not develop it much before four months. Three months is average.

THE PINCER GRASP, EIGHT TO TEN MONTHS. When you pick up a small object between your thumb and forefinger, you are using a pincer grasp. This is a movement of great skill and delicacy for babies. They start using this grasp by about eight or nine months and grow more and more proficient with practice. A few raisins provide a special incentive to master this new skill.

Note: Anything grasped between the thumb and forefinger invariably goes directly to the mouth. Be careful what is lying around for your baby to practice on.

THE TWO-BLOCK TOWER, TWELVE TO EIGHTEEN MONTHS. Between twelve and eighteen months of age, a baby's fine motor coordination has developed to the point where she can pile one block on top of another to form a two-block tower. This key milestone demonstrates eye–hand coordination.

SCRIBBLING ABILITY, TWELVE TO EIGHTEEN MONTHS. A baby can usually hold a crayon in a primitive palmar grasp by one year. The ability to scribble may develop any time after this. Provide crayons to encourage development of this milestone. Supervision is essential—crayons look good enough to eat, and any available surface is as inviting as a blank canvas.

Language Milestones

A baby's first language milestones consist of those noises that only a loving parent can construe as words. Yet these early practice sounds are of vital importance, not because they are a sign of intelligence (they're not), but because their absence may be a sign of a hearing problem. Keep an ear cocked, therefore, for these four key milestones in your baby's language development: babbling, first words, pointing to a named body part, and combining words.

BABBLING, TWO TO SIX MONTHS. A baby begins making rudimentary throat sounds as early as two to six weeks and may be making single sounds, like ga-ga, as early as two to three months. By the time your baby is six or seven months old, she should be babbling with great variations in strength, length, and pitch.

FIRST WORDS, NINE TO TWELVE MONTHS. The first meaningful words are usually either *da-da* or *ma-ma*, and refer to a specific person. The average baby achieves this milestone at about ten months, though some utter their first word as early as nine months, and others not until they are a year old. Of course, da-da and ma-ma may occur much earlier as part of babbling. The key here is if your baby makes the relationship between the word and Mom or Dad.

POINTING TO A NAMED BODY PART, EIGHTEEN TO TWENTY-FOUR MONTHS. Between the ages of eighteen and twenty-four months, the average baby can point to a named body part when prompted ("Show me your leg") and say the word himself. The pronunciation may not be too great— it may come out "weg"—but the meaning should be clear.

COMBINING WORDS, TWENTY TO TWENTY-FOUR MONTHS. The ability to combine words to make sentences is a key milestone that the average child develops at about age twenty months. The first word combinations consist of two-word sentences, such as "Eat lunch" or "Go bed." At twenty-four months, a baby's vocabulary can include as many as three hundred words, and rudimentary conversation begins.

Social Milestones

In their most basic form, social skills can be as elementary as a newborn's fascination with the human face, or a three-year-old's understanding of what it means to take turns. Playing peekaboo is a social milestone, and so is the negativism of the toddler whose favorite new word is "No!" The common denominator that links all of these is the awareness of and interaction with other people. Ultimately, the social milestones your infant attains prepare him to play a healthy and happy role in the human community.

Some key milestones that mark this progress are the social smile, the first games, parallel play, and negativism.

THE SOCIAL SMILE, ONE TO THREE MONTHS. One of the most endearing things a small baby can do is smile. Some observers claim babies smile almost from birth, while others insist these first smiles are little more than random facial movements. Most agree, however, that real facial expressions are evident within the first four to six weeks. Spontaneous smiling develops at about age two months, with some babies starting to do this at six weeks and others not until after twelve weeks. Talking to your baby and smiling at her should be enough to elicit this first social smile.

THE FIRST GAMES, SIX TO EIGHT MONTHS. Real socialization begins sometime between the sixth and eighth months. In this period, a baby will start to enjoy such simple games as peekaboo. They will play these games as long as your patience holds out.

PARALLEL PLAY, EIGHTEEN TO TWENTY-FOUR MONTHS. By the time most infants are one-and-a-half to two years old, they seem to enjoy the company of other babies. They don't yet play together, in the sense of taking turns or sharing toys, but they will play by themselves alongside one another—hence the term *parallel play*. Such play should be supervised at all times.

NEGATIVISM, TWENTY-FOUR TO THIRTY MONTHS. At about the second birthday, toddlers learn a new word and a new concept: "No!" They will say no to every command, and insist on doing things themselves. Frustrating and inconvenient as this may be, it is a sign of your child's developing independence and represents her first attempts to think for herself.

CHAPTER 15

PARENTING

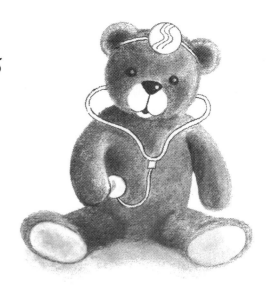

The noun *parent* is an old word that we all use easily, but the verb *to parent* and its derivative *parenting* expand on the older concept of being a parent to include many more things. Parenting is more than mothering because it includes the very important function of fathering, as well. Fathers are now regularly involved with their children from their presence in the birthing room to a greater sharing of responsibility for all aspects of the baby's care at home.

Parenting is more than nurturing, because it requires more than providing nourishment, shelter, encouragement, and support. It implies intelligent decision making, the ability to participate in your child's health care, awareness of environmental dangers, and willingness to appreciate your child as an individual; it also includes all of the many other intangibles that go with the experience and responsibility of being in charge of someone else's life.

It sounds awesome. Actually, it is a loving, fulfilling experience, and great fun, once you learn to relax and enjoy it.

Most of this book has been about one major aspect of parenting—your part in monitoring the health, growth, and development of your baby. Since it is impossible to include everything about parenting in one book, let alone one chapter, we will discuss just five other aspects of parenting here that bear most closely on the physical and emotional health of infants and toddlers: parent–child bonding, parent–child relationship, guidance and discipline, feeding and nutrition, and accident prevention.

Parent-Child Bonding

The bond that forms between parents and a new baby is one of the most important and one of the strongest of human relationships. Scientifically speaking, this bond is a survival mechanism that assures the baby of food, protection, and good prospects for achieving adulthood as a functioning member of society. In many ways, parent-child bonding is comparable to the nesting and protective instincts of other animals, except that it is carried to a higher degree in humans, and we call it love. When this bond fails to develop or breaks down for some reason, a baby's health may be at considerable risk. Feeding may not be as it should be, hygienic care may be haphazard, the child can be emotionally distressed as a result of rejection, and in extreme cases the baby may be subjected to overt physical abuse.

Because the development of a strong parent-child bond is so important to a baby's health, doctors have become interested in learning just how the bond forms. There are no definitive answers yet, but studies done so far have resulted in some interesting observations.

Mothers seem to experience a state of heightened sensitivity, which lasts for a few weeks after giving birth, and close contact between mother and baby during this period seems to enhance the quality of the bond that develops between them. Doctors who have become interested in the bonding experience usually recommend intimate private contact between mother and baby in the hours immediately after birth, and then as much as possible every day for the first few weeks. If, because of medical problems, the baby has to be kept in the hospital nursery after birth, arrangements are usually made for the parents to see and fondle the baby as much as his condition will allow.

In several studies, the following advantages were noted during the first three years of life when mothers had an opportunity for close contact with their babies in the first hours and days after birth:

- Mothers showed more affection for their babies.

- Mothers spent more time with their babies.

- Mothers used more words talking to babies, but fewer imperatives.

- The period of breast-feeding was generally longer.

- There were fewer home accidents.

- There were fewer mothering disorders.

Parent-child bonding probably begins to develop during pregnancy and is enhanced by certain landmark events—when the mother first feels signs of life; when the father is able to feel movement in the mother's womb or hear the baby's heartbeat; and when the father and mother pore over lists of names and fantasize over the appearance and future of their unborn baby. Immediately after the baby is born, doctors and nurses have observed a pattern of behavior when a mother is presented with her new baby. It is clearly part of the bonding process and progresses as follows:

- Mother examines the baby with her fingertips. She will usually touch fingers and toes first.

- In a few minutes, mother begins to rub the baby with her whole hand.

- Baby and mother lie face-to-face and establish eye contact.

- Baby reaches out and makes sounds; arms move forward, the head moves back, the pupils of the eyes dilate, and the face brightens.

- Baby will grasp mother's finger if it is presented; if not, baby grasps anything handy—his shirt or gown if he is wearing one.

- There is a peak of excitement for both mother and baby, and then both calm down. Their emotions seem to be synchronized. Baby may avert his eyes and mother may feel like relaxing.

Fathers also have a bonding experience, although men are more subject to cultural influences in how they are expected to act. A rather typical action profile goes like this:

- Father looks at the child and admires its many fine features.

- If it's a first baby, father may be concerned about small imperfections. He should be reassured about things that will straighten themselves out in a short time.

- There is an urge to touch the baby and hold it. This should be encouraged since new fathers often wait for permission to touch and fondle a newborn.

- Father perceives the baby as his own. He focuses attention on characteristics that might be like his own.

- There is a feeling of self-esteem and satisfaction; extreme pleasure and elation.

- Baby heightens the experience of bonding with his grasp reflex and visual alertness. He apparently takes an instant liking to Dad, grasping his finger when it is invariably presented.

Strong bonding carries parents through the difficult times of parenting, and creates a positive attitude that ensures baby's physical and emotional well-being. Where a high-quality bond exists— where there is love, in other words—baby is virtually assured of high-quality care and guidance.

Not all mothers, however, fall in love with their babies instantly, especially if labor and delivery have been difficult and high levels of sedation have been necessary. In nearly all cases, however, bonding does occur within the first week. In an instance where a mother is forced to be separated from her baby in the early days or in the case of adoptive parents, bonding occurs later and in slightly different ways. But it does occur, and you shouldn't feel guilty if feelings of love are delayed for some reason. In the few cases where parents have doubts about their feelings, they should seek professional counseling without delay.

The Parent-Child Relationship

From the moment of birth, a baby perceives the world almost entirely in terms of parents and other caregivers. Whether the world is seen by your infant as safe and nurturing, or painful and hostile depends entirely on you and on others who have contact with her. And to some extent, children continue to see the world as their parents do well into their teen years, even though it may not seem so in those later, trying times. If you treat your child with love and respect, chances are excellent you will raise your child to be a loving and considerate adult. If you place confidence in your child, within the limits of her development, you may expect to send an independent, self-confident person into the world when home ties are finally broken. If you are hostile, domineering, belligerent, abusive, or fearful, chances are just as good that you will find similar negative characteristics in your child.

The process for establishing a good relationship with your baby is based on common good sense and some very obvious attitudes—such as regarding your child as a fellow human with feelings just like your own, as a person requiring the same love and respect that you require yourself. Many parents proceed along these lines instinctively, usually because they have been brought up this way themselves; but others have to shed old notions about the need for harsh and thoughtless discipline, which they mistake for guidance, because that's how it was when they were growing up.

Don't fall into the trap of believing that a child doesn't feel the way you do because she can't express herself the way you do. Babies do suffer from poor relationships with their parents, even if they can't tell you about it.

The expression "failure to thrive" is used to describe children who don't grow as they should, may be sickly, and lag in developing motor and mental skills. There are two categories of failure to thrive: one category is physical or organic, where some body system is not working as it should because of a defect or a disease condition; the other category of failure to thrive is a result of the child's psychological and social environment, often referred to as "parent deprivation." In this case, the child is neglected or abused—physically or mentally—by a misguided or uncaring parent.

We tend to think of parent deprivation as occurring only in poor socioeconomic situations. This is not the case. It can occur wherever parents are under stress—emotional, financial, or social. Family stress, of course, is unavoidable in the best of situations. But if you have taken pains to establish a good relationship with your child, from infancy onward, everyone will survive the occasional storms without major damage. Here, in summary, are some of the most important precepts for establishing a good relationship with infants and older children:

1. *A child needs a safe, nurturing environment in which to grow.* This refers to the basics you provide: a nutritious diet; a warm, comfortable place; security; comfort; love; and caring. An infant develops a sense of trust very early, but only if it has reason to trust. An orderly routine, consistency of care, and reasonable rules and expectations are included here as well.

2. *Relax and enjoy your child.* Everything works better when you are relaxed. A parent who calculates every move and frets over what she may be doing wrong will communicate her fearfulness to the child. If you are tense, an infant's prolonged crying can make you frantic; a two-year-old's temper tantrum can put you in a panic; persistent disobedience can send you into a rage. If you are under profound stress, you should seek professional help. Arrange for a short vacation from your child if you need one.

3. *You can't give your child too much love.* People need love and wither without it. If you can't do anything else right except provide your baby with love, he will probably do pretty well for himself. Some people feel they lose status and respect if they display affection. This is usually a cultural thing. Don't be afraid to hug, kiss, and touch. It's good for baby and it's good for you. It will strengthen your position of authority rather than diminish it, because when your child loves and respects you, your simple disapproval will carry more weight than a spanking. Loving, incidentally, is a lifelong ingredient of good parenting that is prescribed for grown children as well as for cuddly new babies.

4. *You can't spoil a baby with love and indulgence.* This is a corollary of the proposition that you can't give too much love. It doesn't mean that you must give a baby or a child everything he

wants or allow any kind of behavior. But it doesn't hurt to pick up a fretting infant instead of letting him "cry it out." If a baby plasters himself and his surroundings with cereal, you might stop to think if he will learn more from the plastering or from a slap on the hands. Be sure you know the difference between "bad" behavior and normal childish behavior that you find annoying or embarrassing. Indulgence, as we use it here, means giving baby the benefit of the doubt where the motives for his behavior are concerned. Don't assume he is being bad until you think it through, which is probably the way you wish your own behavior to be evaluated.

5. *You are your child's role model.* Children are great mimics. It's how they learn to be people. They observe you even when you think they don't notice or don't understand what is going on. It is probably too much to ask that a person give up all bad habits upon becoming a parent, but it is a good idea to reevaluate the worst of them if you don't want them to become a part of your child's personality. You might want to give up smoking, for example, so that your child won't copy this unhealthy habit.

6. *Provide learning experiences for your child.* Having a baby does not mean that you must give up your own life. It is self-defeating in the long run to give all of your time and effort to your child (or children) because, in most cases, parents come to resent such a sacrifice and then may come to resent the child herself. The important thing is that time spent with your child be quality time. An hour's reading together or a walk in the park that you both enjoy thoroughly is worth far more than a

cranky day at the zoo that makes you both miserable. Provide appropriate play opportunities. Mobiles and crib toys are an important learning experience for an infant. Later, pots and pans, putting things into other things, experimenting with sounds and textures, touching, tasting, trying are all part of learning about the world and one's place in it. Speak to your child; you can't start too early to give your baby language experience. Give her picture books. Have magazines available that can be played with and destroyed as baby wishes. Make reading fun, and show by your own example that it is something everybody does.

7. *Be informed.* You should know what to expect in the way of behavior at various stages in your baby's life. When you are informed, you will be more likely to understand why an eight-month-old will suddenly start crying when left alone and why a two-year-old may be stubbornly negative. It is frustrating for you and potentially damaging to your child when you misunderstand and punish normal behavior as being "bad" or "spoiled."

Read a number of books on child behavior. Ask friends which books they have found most useful, then buy two or three favorites for home reference. You have to be cautious in your reading, however. Fads come and go, philosophies differ, and some "experts" have dubious qualifications. Every parent-child relationship is unique and you should not feel obliged to follow every new revelation in the popular press.

If your child has a special problem—a chronic ailment, a disability, stuttering, learning difficulties—seek out literature about the problem. Contact the appropriate organizations that provide support and information about your problem. Find professional, specialized help when it is needed.

Guidance and Discipline (Infants to Four Years)

In many Asian and indigenous American cultures, children are pampered and indulged, but they are also provided with guidance and taught the disciplines considered acceptable in their cultures. Guidance is equated with teaching—usually by example—and discipline suggests control, as in self-control, and setting behavioral guidelines that are not to be exceeded.

In our own society, we seem to go through phases in our understanding of guidance and discipline. In one era, our idea of guidance and discipline is expressed as "spare the rod and spoil the child," which implies teaching through beating, the most self-defeating idea ever conjured up by supposedly civilized people. In another era, complete permissiveness becomes the fashion, leaving children hungering for the guidance and direction they need as they progress through developmental stages. Guidance and discipline, used in the proper sense, serve each other. Punishment is only a part of discipline, and the best punishment teaches a positive lesson rather than a negative one.

In controlling discipline, the trick is in understanding the difference between misbehavior—being bad—and the behavioral stages a child goes through for good reason. You have to develop appropriate responses to expected behavior just as you respond to other aspects of growth. Your responses to your child's behavior are, in effect, the guidance and discipline you offer him; and they should be undertaken with the same love and con-

cern for your child's growth and development that you give to his physical well-being.

The following pages offer a review of child behavior from infancy through the preschool years. It is not by any means comprehensive, but it does tell you, in general, what to expect, and it also provides suggestions for appropriate responses. For more detailed information about child behavior, read one of the many excellent books on the subject. If you find yourself always spanking, nagging, and punishing your child, and utterly distracted by his behavior, it may be well to seek help from a qualified psychologist or family guidance counselor.

Never discipline a child or vent your anger by shaking. Shaking can result in irreversible brain damage from intracranial bleeding. When shaken baby syndrome is discovered by a doctor it is reportable as a child abuse felony.

Infants—Birth to Six Months

An infant is completely dependent on parents and other caregivers, and she learns from them that the new environment is one where she can be safe. Though baby is nonverbal, parents soon learn to read her body language and understand the meanings of various sounds she makes. Baby responds to adults' verbal and nonverbal behavior—sounds, stroking, patting, and cuddling. Maintaining body contact is comforting, and most kinds of gentle movements are enjoyed. Infants are repelled and frightened by loud sounds and rough handling. A stranger (even a grandparent) who swoops down on an infant, albeit with the best of intentions, will set off a frightened howl.

DEVELOPMENTAL PLAY. Moving baby's arms and legs, touching fingers and toes (this little piggy), and gentle pokes are all fun. Baby likes color and movement in crib toys, tinkling sounds, clock ticking, soft music, and singing. It's never too early to talk to him. He likes the sound of your voice and eventually will start to make sense of the sounds.

PROBLEMS. Crying and fussing are the big problems at this age. A fretful, colicky baby is especially difficult. Hunger, fear, pain, body restraint, loneliness, and boredom can all cause crying. Most of the time, you can quickly rule out illness (you have seen how to do this in earlier chapters), and you can check for obvious things like a skin irritation. Feeding, carrying, comforting, motion of any kind, singing, music are all good to try. If your baby is particularly difficult and illness has been ruled out by the doctor, you must learn to get along with her as best you can, secure in the knowledge that things will get better. Enlist loving relatives and friends to relieve you once in a while.

DISCIPLINE. Any sort of punishment or attempts at discipline make no sense at this age; it is counterproductive, in fact. Leaving baby to "cry it out" is likely to drive you up a wall and won't accomplish anything. Accommodate yourself to baby's needs. If movement or company quiets your baby in a difficult time, put her in a portable crib that you can rock with your toe as you read; or keep her nearby so you can talk to her as you work.

Babies—Six to Twelve Months

Baby is beginning to develop likes and dislikes; mood swings are wide and often unexplainable. Baby may cuddle and kiss one minute and be howling with anger the next. He begins to show fears— of strangers, of being left alone, of the dark, of going to bed.

DEVELOPMENTAL PLAY. Baby is grasping and manipulating things by six months and experimenting with her senses—feeling, tasting, turning toward sounds, and showing great visual interest in events around her. All this increases as she stands and begins to find means of moving about. Provide things of different sizes and textures for her to play with. She will discover the joy of dropping toys on the floor, which will provide you with great exercise for your abdominal muscles and hamstrings as you bend to pick them up. Avoid the temptation to tie toys to the crib or playpen with string. Strings, even short ones, can be dangerous.

PROBLEMS. Separation anxiety sets in around six to eight months. When mother and father are gone, they have ceased to exist as far as the baby is concerned, and he howls. Return and comfort the baby. Play peekaboo games to show that you reappear after disappearing briefly. Call from the next room to show that you are there.

Stranger anxiety is related to separation anxiety. The baby is suddenly suspicious of all strangers (including grandparents) and rejects most people. This is normal behavior. People should not reach for the baby or swoop down on him. If the baby must be left with a sitter, introduce the sitter gradually. Stay around until the baby is quite used to the new person. Then withdraw gradually once he is comfortable and feels secure.

The baby may be frightened in the dark by shadows or noises. Provide comfort and reassurance. It doesn't hurt to leave a small night-light on. By six months, most babies will sleep through the night, but for many, sleep becomes a problem. Advice from pediatricians range from letting a wakeful baby "cry it out" to taking the child to bed with you. A compromise position is probably better. Some babies will quiet down with soft music.

A little gentle rubbing and talking to until sleep returns may work. Like other problems, waiting for your baby to establish a better sleep pattern may simply take patience. It will happen, and in the meantime you will probably find that giving in promotes more family harmony than toughing it out in a combat of wills with an infant.

Mood changes, likes, and dislikes are hard to understand in a small baby. Realize that the baby is a person who is subject to moods, likes, and dislikes, just as you are. If the baby decides not to like some food, try another. If he is grouchy, try to talk him out of it or leave him alone. The next mood will be along shortly. He may dislike being washed, changed, and fussed with. Do what you have to do anyhow in a matter-of-fact way and with as much good will as possible.

DISCIPLINE. A baby still cannot understand punishment at this age; when attempted it makes matters worse. Do things you have to do with confidence and dispatch, even though she objects. Keep as regular a routine as you can so she knows what to expect. This, in effect, is teaching discipline as the baby comes to know there are things that must and will be done.

Toddlers—Twelve to Thirty Months

This period includes the "terrible twos" and the "terrible no" stages. The toddler is fully mobile and off adventuring. He is into everything, and consequently he is a danger to everything in the house, including himself. He seems accident prone. In his driving for autonomy, he will test you and your limits as well as his own. He will be stubborn, negative, and obstinate. He has the fears and mood swings of a younger child and, if anything, they

are intensified. He can't make fine distinctions between what is a good thing to do and what is a bad thing. If you can turn over a toy chest, why not a garbage can? Mealtime is often turned into playtime, messing about in the food, standing, and experimenting with dishes and utensils. But it gives you something to look forward to—age three when this behavior seems to stop as suddenly as it started. And through it all, intense learning has been going on.

DEVELOPMENTAL PLAY. The best procedure is to clear the decks for action. Anything you don't want touched must go out-of-sight or out-of-reach. Some parents leave things at child level that are okay to play with. They provide a low drawer or closet filled with things baby can take in and out to her heart's content—pots, rags, empty boxes, a few toys. Toddlers like things they can push and pull, and toys should be simple. They often prefer the box a present came in to the present itself. Anything that makes noise when you shake it is grand; anything that can be put in, taken out, or banged on provides endless enjoyment. But a toddler won't see the difference between banging a pot with a spoon or banging your glass coffee table with a hammer. There is no sex difference in preferences for toys. Boys are fond of dolls, girls will dig in dirt. Don't expect them to play your way. A toddler will not always run a train on tracks, color within the lines, or work a dress-up doll properly. Don't try to change her methods.

PROBLEMS. Remove dangerous and valuable objects from her path; this is preferable to following her around, slapping her hands, and saying, "Don't." Some things can't be moved, of course, so the toddler can't be left alone for a minute.

Remember she is a danger to herself as well as to your valuables. Remove her and interest her in something safe. If she's after a hot stove, warn her, "The stove will hurt you." Choose your words carefully. Warning her that it is "hot," a concept she may not know, often leads to her going after the stove again saying, "hot, hot" with great delight. Don't bother with warnings about future behavior such as "Don't touch Grandma's cups." She might not have thought of it if you hadn't made the suggestion, and she won't grasp the notion of consequences if she goes ahead anyway.

No is a fascinating new word. It is used by baby to test her autonomy and your limits. Counter this by not asking questions when you don't really want your baby to make a choice. Instead of asking, "Would you like to take a nap?", announce that it is nap time. To avoid scenes, announce an order of events in advance: "After the story, it's bedtime." "Put the dolly to bed and then come and eat lunch."

Toddlers at this age are quick to anger and to screaming rages. If removing a child from something he is doing sends him into a temper, carry through as gracefully as you can without anger. Be consistent in enforcing limits. There is no reasoning with a temper tantrum, and a slap or yelling won't stop it. Let it play out, and carry through with your plans. As the tantrum subsides, comfort and reassure the child. He may even hold his breath to the point of unconsciousness. But he will breathe again automatically. Tantrums are shattering experiences, but they are more survivable if you stay calm.

Thumb sucking usually peaks at eighteen or twenty months. It's not a problem to worry about. It won't bother the teeth until the permanent set starts to erupt, about age six, and by that time chances are the child will have stopped. If you object to thumb sucking, you may prefer to offer a pacifier. Don't use restraints or bad-tasting medicines on the thumb. If the child is an inveterate thumb sucker and is also listless and apathetic, call this to the doctor's attention.

Shadows, ghosts, unexplainable things (one child called them "hmm-hms") can frighten a child. These are legitimate fears for a baby, and she should be reassured and comforted. Don't punish a two-year-old by putting her in a dark room or a closet. Leave her bedroom door open and a light on if she prefers. Halloween masks, clowns, and pumpkins can send a small child into paroxysms of terror. Avoid a trick-or-treat night until the child is ready for it. Don't force a child to touch a dog if she is afraid of dogs. Let her watch others playing with the dog until she's sure it is safe. Don't force a child to do anything that seems to frighten her. She'll be brave soon enough.

Toddlers are often picky and may reject a whole meal because of one thing they don't like. You may catch your child in a "mood" at mealtime, either fussy or ready to play and experiment, and, of course, either one will make feeding difficult. Offer small portions and go back for more if he is eating well. If he rejects a food, it is easier to try an equally nutritious substitute than to fight over it. Avoid caving in completely, offering potato chips and cookies because "he has to have something." Feeding games often work—"open the door so the plane can fly in." Uncovering the bunny on the bottom of the dish sometimes creates interest. (But see the cautions about overfeeding in the next section.) If your best efforts seem useless, give up and he'll be hungrier for the next meal.

DISCIPLINE. Remove a toddler from dangerous or destructive situations with a stern word of disapproval. On the other hand, be effusive with your praise when she is doing something acceptable. Even if it doesn't seem like anything to brag about, admire the way she plays with the pots or pulls a toy.

A toddler tends to go into his worst moods at the worst possible times—when you are exhausted, as you are leaving for a rare night out, as friends arrive for a dinner party. Try to anticipate such problems and insist that the baby proceed with his own routine regardless of his nasty mood. If you have a competent babysitter for your night out, steel yourself and go. If you are exhausted, turn the baby over to your spouse or arrange for an occasional sitter to give you a respite even if you are home. Hire a sitter when you are entertaining. The point is, baby's life should be conducted in a consistent and orderly manner, and he must learn that he can't manipulate you with his moods.

When punishing, make the punishment fit the crime and do it quickly before the child forgets what she has done. If baby is drawing on the walls with crayons after she has been shown that this is unacceptable behavior, take away the crayons. Be sure that both parents share the responsibility of disciplining, so that one parent does not become the heavy. Whenever you can, try to avoid punishment by heading off trouble you can see coming.

For those times when nothing but physical aggression will suffice to vent your feelings, kick a hassock or a door. Your child will get the point as clearly as if you had aimed one at her.

A Summary of Toddler Discipline

1. Set reasonable limits and insist upon them firmly and consistently. The toddler must learn what is dangerous, destructive, and unacceptable. Try not to limit harmless activities; baby should have some privileges as a member of the family.

2. Praise good and acceptable behavior. Most children will try hard to please.

3. Allow for accidents.

4. Make the punishment fit the crime. Don't overdo it. Shutting a child up in the dark, slapping, taking away a favorite teddy bear or blanket may be too strong for a toddler to handle.

5. Toddlers prefer structure, routine, and consistency. They find laissez-faire confusing. If you have to change a routine, try to do it gradually, allowing for baby's natural conservatism.

6. Toddlers are too young to reason with. Avoid detailed explanations. Be simple, direct, and positive. At the same time be friendly and good natured about your directions. Watch your tone and attitude.

7. Be sure baby understands you love him. Once resolved, conflicts can be put behind with a hug. Make baby a part of your life and activities whenever possible. Help and encourage her to explore, experiment, and seek for autonomy in safe and acceptable ways. This is what she really wants and what her cantankerous and contrary behavior is making her strive for.

Preschool Children—Three to Four Years

Most parents look back on this period as the best time in their children's lives, and the one they enjoyed the most. Though he is still a baby in many ways, you may suddenly discover that your child has become more of a companion. He talks, gets about easily, plays recognizable games, loves to be read to, is toilet trained, and has mastered a good deal of self-care. He can join in a meal as one of the family.

It is an age of discovery, inventiveness, and intense learning. Many of the "cute" things you will remember with pleasure come out of this period. But a preschooler is still learning proper behavior, which means you can't expect 100 percent success.

PROBLEMS. A preschooler talks incessantly, is very curious, and constantly asks, "Why?" But she wants simple, direct answers rather than long explanations. She understands more words than she can speak, so be careful of what you say in front of her, thinking she won't understand. A preschooler will surely embarrass you by repeating street words. Just explain that these are words the family doesn't use, and you would rather not hear them. Avoid a fuss over this harmless experimentation.

Your preschooler may still have baby fears of the dark and of going to bed alone. Work on these slowly, never forcing or shaming her. She may still be timid about strangers and about anything that seems dangerous to her. But unlike the two-year-old, she can adapt to a new situation easily if it is explained in advance and introduced slowly. If you have to leave a preschooler at a day-care center, for instance, it will be easier if she has seen the place and the people beforehand, if you have explained the situation to her, and if she is allowed to take some of her familiar things with her—a toy, a book, or a security blanket.

Nursery school is generally a good idea for preschoolers if the care is good and the leaders make the experience a positive one. Nursery school provides a group experience and excellent stimulation for physical, social, and language development. Prepare your child well in advance, however. Pay casual visits to the facility and watch the children play. When he starts nursery school, spend the first session or two with him until you are certain he fits into the group and the supervision is stimulating and competent. Provide the teacher or other caretaker with detailed information about your child's likes and dislikes, fears, names of siblings and pets, terms used for going to the toilet, and any other things the teacher will need to know to make your child feel comfortable in the new situation. (When the school requests this information, it is a clue to their awareness and competence.)

DEVELOPMENTAL PLAY. Preschoolers engage in parallel play with other children and in cooperative play. Parallel play occurs when children play together but each follows his or her own course—such as when children sit in a sandbox together and each works with her own pail and shovel. Cooperative play occurs when children get together, plan their activity, and assign roles.

You are likely to find your preschooler talking to imaginary playmates; this is normal, and he will do this less and less as he plays with other children more and more. It is also a great time for imitating. Children this age love to clop around in parents' shoes and play at doing things they see you and older siblings doing. They like to "help," imitating you as you do household chores.

This is a period where your child is using a larger variety of playthings than he had before or will again. He needs playground equipment for running, jumping, and climbing. He will use rudimentary sports equipment, a sandbox, wading pool, trucks, wagons, and a sled in winter. He likes picture books, easy construction sets and crafts, and paints and crayons. There isn't much he won't play with, in fact, if he can even begin to manage it.

DISCIPLINE. Your preschooler wants guidance and wants to be very clear about the limits you set on behavior. Be firm and consistent about this. Because a preschooler wants so badly to please her parents, she can be crushed very easily. Don't mock or shame her. She is very literal and doesn't understand teasing too well.

Don't make threats that you don't intend to carry out. If punishment is necessary it should be immediate, it should fit the crime, and it should never be more severe than the child can handle. Be sure to make up when it is all behind you.

REGRESSION. Regression is a return to behavior that a child had clearly put behind him some months or even years before. A toilet-trained child may begin soiling again; a three-year-old may start using a sibling's nursing bottle or throw temper tantrums like a two-year-old. A toddler may suddenly "forget" how to walk, or a preschooler may use baby talk or cease talking altogether.

Regression can occur at times of stress for the child. Severe illness, a hospital stay, separation from parents, a drastic change in routine, a new caretaker, the arrival of a new brother or sister, may create enough stress to make the child seek the security of an earlier age.

Regressive behavior often frightens or angers parents. It usually happens at the worst possible time, when parents themselves are experiencing the same difficult situation the child is. The best approach to regression is to make as little of it as you can, once you assure yourself that illness is not the cause of the problem. Comfort and reassure

your child to help her through the stressful time. Praise whatever she is still doing right. If the regressive behavior persists or becomes too much for you to handle, seek professional help. If the stress is obviously caused by the arrival of a sibling, consult one of the many good books on child behavior that make suggestions for dealing with this situation.

Feeding and Nutrition

Breast-Feeding

If a mother is willing and capable of breast-feeding, it is unanimously agreed today that it is best for both mother and baby. There are really only two reasons why a mother can't breast-feed: one is if the mother has a serious, debilitating illness and the other is if the baby has a lactose deficiency and is unable to digest natural milk. Even in cases of mastitis (inflammation of the breast), most doctors will suggest it is better to continue nursing while the mother is being treated, unless it is just too painful to carry on.

These are the benefits of breast-feeding:

- Breast-feeding helps the bonding process between mother and child.

- Breast milk is the most perfect food for infants.

- Breast-feeding is economical and convenient—no bottles to prepare, no formula to buy, and the milk is always available at the correct temperature, free of contamination.

- Breast-fed babies usually do not overfeed and, consequently, do not overgain.

- Constipation is rare in breast-fed babies; colic, spitting up, and allergies are less common.

- Breast milk, especially colostrum, which is the first fluid before true milk comes in, contains antibodies against several of the common viruses and bacteria. Breast-fed babies tend to have fewer respiratory infections during the first year of life.

- Breast-feeding stimulates contraction of the uterus.

- Mothers who breast-feed have a lower incidence of breast cancer.

Clearly, you must want to nurse before you will find the experience beneficial and satisfying. If a mother is not emotionally ready for breast-feeding, chances are she will not be very successful at it. National, cultural, social, and class differences may influence your decision to breast-feed or not. Because the decision must be made soon after the baby is born, think about it during pregnancy. There are many good books on the subject, and veteran nursing mothers will be glad to give you the benefit of their experiences. Your doctor will advise, of course, and can direct you to a local chapter of La Leche League and can tell you how to get information and videos from the American Academy of Pediatrics.

As stated, the first material secreted by the mother's breast is colostrum, a slightly cloudy fluid that contains important nutrients for your baby plus the antibodies mentioned earlier. Babies are routinely put to the breast in the birthing room whenever possible, or as soon after birth as is practical, when they are calm and seem willing to do some serious sucking.

Production of "true" milk begins within a day or sometimes within a few days of your baby's birth. Such a delay is normal and no supplementation with formula is necesary. During the first few weeks, the baby should be only breast-fed in order to encourage optimal milk production, but after that an occasional supplemental bottle can be introduced, preferably given by someone besides the mother—the father, for example. This is so that mother can have some freedom from time to time, and the baby can get used to someone else holding and feeding her. Many nursing mothers express their own milk from their breasts for this purpose and save it in the refrigerator, or in the freezer if it's not to be used soon. Otherwise formula milk is used.

One thing is clear: in order to do a good job of nursing, a mother must start with a positive attitude, be relaxed about it, and enjoy it. Mothers who don't want to nurse or who find it objectionable are usually poor milk producers. Mothers who enjoy breast-feeding usually nurse their babies more frequently, and frequent nursing encourages milk flow. Good diet and adequate fluid intake also help assure quality milk production. Some drugs and other substances can appear in mothers' milk in undesirable quantities, so be sure to check with your doctor if you are taking medication, either prescribed or nonprescribed.

Formula Feeding

Formula feeding via a nursing bottle is a much more complicated procedure than breast-feeding. You can make formula yourself from scratch (an involved procedure involving recipes, equipment, and precise measuring), or as most parents do, you can choose from a variety of commercial products that have a cow's-milk base or a soy base. They are available in powder form to be mixed with water or in cans ready-mixed and ready to use.

Opinions vary about which of the various formula options to use. Cost, convenience, your doctor's preferences, and the baby's constitution all influence your decision. Inform yourself about the options while you are pregnant and discuss them with your doctor. Not all babies thrive on the same feeding, and sometimes it takes a bit of fine-tuning before you and your doctor find a formula that works best for your baby.

Whatever the formula, feed your baby as though you were breast-feeding. Cuddle him close, rock him gently and speak soothingly. Mother–child bonding takes place with formula-fed babies as well as with breast-fed babies, but the quality of the bond is usually better if you work at it a bit.

Weaning and Solid Food

In years gone by, early weaning was considered by some mothers to be a sign of sophistication. Thus, many children were started on solid food at two months or even younger. This is not a good idea because an infant's digestive system is really not prepared to handle anything except mother's milk or properly designed formula until four months at the earliest. The conventional wisdom today is to wait until six months to start solid food, or until the baby weighs twelve or thirteen pounds. The digestive system is better prepared for it, the baby is beginning to show signs of teeth, and she may be ready to make a first attempt at drinking from a cup.

Work out a timetable for switching from breast-feeding and formula feeding to cow's milk with your doctor. Whole milk is usually recommended for children up to age two because the fat is needed for growth and development. There can be reasons for making other choices, however, and this should be discussed with your doctor.

Iron-fortified infant cereal is usually the first supplement introduced to your baby's diet. Mix the cereal with baby's formula or with diluted cow's milk. At first, she will only take one or two spoonfuls. Keep offering cereal on a spoon twice a day until the baby learns to recognize the spoon and has developed her chewing and swallowing mechanisms to handle the new form of eating. Don't force it. Keep mealtimes pleasant and fun, and the baby will learn how to handle solid foods quickly enough. The first spoonfuls will invariably be spit or dribbled back out, not because the baby doesn't like the food or is being stubborn. Sucking involves thrusting the tongue forward and the baby will try to eat the new food in the same way she sucks milk from the breast or bottle. Just scrape the cereal off her chin and try again as long as she is willing.

Once the baby has learned to take infant cereal, other foods can be added one at a time. When you try foods one at a time, you can get a better idea of baby's preferences. You will probably have more success if you introduce fruits and vegetables before meat, but the order of introducing new foods is not important.

Commercial strained foods should probably be used first, simply because it is easier and you can be sure you are feeding foods proved to be acceptable to babies. After your baby has learned to eat a variety of strained foods, you may prefer to cook and strain fresh products, but it is important to remember his kidneys are immature and have limited salt-excreting capability. Therefore, avoid adding either sugar or salt when you prepare infant food at home.

Once the baby is taking solid foods, he should be taught to drink from a cup. His water needs will increase at this time, and he may fuss when he is thirsty. It is important that water be offered in other ways besides milk. Apple juice, orange juice, and plain water can be given. Bottles of juice should not be used as a pacifier at this point, however. Teeth are beginning to erupt, and the sugar and acids in juices promote tooth decay when they are allowed to stay in contact with the teeth for as long as it takes to drink a bottle. Avoid highly sugared drinks and soda.

After your baby has grown a few teeth, chopped foods can be introduced. Then, once molars have appeared, usually by age two, children can eat regular table foods.

Eating and Overeating

A complete discussion of nutrition is far beyond the scope of this book, but the following must be said because it is so important: a fat baby is not necessarily a healthy baby. Overeating (and the resulting obesity), possibly the most serious health problem in developed nations, often is a result of poor eating habits established for children by their parents in their first months and years of life.

Both overeating and genetics are factors in the development of obesity, so just as adults in families that tend to obesity have special problems in controlling their weight, children of obese parents have a harder row to hoe than children of lean parents. If one parent is substantially overweight, a child has a 40 percent chance of being obese. If both parents are substantially overweight, a child has more than a 70 percent chance of becoming

obese. So when a child's genetic history marks her as a candidate for becoming overweight, parents should make a special effort to give her a good start in her eating habits. Although some overweight children occasionally do slim out in later years, it is more often true that obese children become obese adults. Therefore, parents should make every effort to keep their children lean, though not undernourished, of course.

At five or six months, a baby indicates he wants food by opening his mouth and leaning forward. He indicates that he is full or disinterested in food by leaning back and away from the food and turning his head. When that happens, don't force the issue. Let him control it. Similarly, don't coax a bottle-fed baby to take more than he wants. (Breast-fed babies are usually in better control of their eating than bottle-fed babies whose mothers tend to coax them to finish the last drop of prescribed formula.) By teaching your child to overeat early in life, you may be setting the stage for a lifelong battle with obesity.

If your child does begin to become obese, it is not necessary for him to lose weight, but simply not to gain for a while. Allow his growth to catch up with his weight. Cut back on high-calorie foods, particularly fats and starches, and encourage low-calorie, high-bulk foods like vegetables. Once your child is obese and has developed the specialized cells necessary to hold and store fat, it is much harder for him to lose weight than it would have been had he not developed the fat storage cells in the first place. It is also far easier to regain lost weight after an abundance of fat storage cells have developed. For those adults familiar with the battle of the bulge, this is old news.

Actually, enough has been said on this subject that every reasonable parent knows that snacks should consist of fruit slices or foods such as graham crackers and milk. Why, then, are babies still overfed? The following are some of your most formidable adversaries (you might want to add a few of your own to the list):

- Television ads for heavily sugared snacks, cereals, and drinks

- Frequent trips to fast-food restaurants for french fries and shakes

- Doting relatives who use sweets to show baby they love her

- Parents and relatives who are culturally acclimated to forcing a child to eat

- Parent role models who have horrible eating and snacking habits themselves

- Fast-heat-'em-and-eat-'em dinners that are mostly starch, fat, sugar, salt, and chemicals.

An easy trick that can revolutionize your toddler's or preschooler's diet is to keep a precise record of everything she eats for one week. If you don't conclude that she is getting too much of the wrong things, you are a very unusual parent indeed.

Protecting Your Child— Physical Needs

It goes without saying that an important part of parenting consists of providing a home for your baby that is clean, snug, and safe, where baby can grow and develop with a reasonable feeling of regularity and security in his life. Baby should have a place to sleep that is quiet and safe for him, and have adequate clothes to keep him comfortable and looking nice.

Though we take these things for granted, it's sometimes easier said than done. Housing is costly,

and many young couples must start out in old buildings where there may be problems with heat, cleanliness, or aspects of safety. Clothing is outrageously expensive, and many a tight budget buckles under the cost of a tiny pair of shoes. It all takes a great deal of work and careful planning. It can also be fun, however. Providing a safe home and attractive clothing and furnishings for a new baby is as imporant for your own morale and sense of parenthood as it is necessary for baby's comfort.

Clothing and Furnishings

You won't lack help in deciding what a new baby needs in the way of clothing and furniture. The problem is more likely to be how to get and pay for it all. Don't be bashful about letting your needs be known. People like to know what gifts you want. Make lists and check off items as they are acquired. Unless you have a large income, go secondhand for the things you have to buy yourself. Let your friends with older children know you are happy to receive hand-me-downs. Many families have favorite clothing go through six or more children. When you are through with clothing, pass it on to others.

Tag sales (garage sales), upscale charity retail outlets, and well-run private secondhand stores are all good bets for better-quality clothes and furnishings than you might be able to afford otherwise. Bargains in baby furniture abound in classified ads. Don't get the foolish notion that you're turning baby into a "Secondhand Rose." You can find secondhand woolens, linens, and corduroys that cost far less than cheap acrylics in discount stores. Have the clothes cleaned (though they will have been cleaned already if they're from a good source) and personalize them with monograms or ready-made appliqués from a fabric store.

A crib and chest of drawers you refinish yourself can have more meaning than a slick new set you get off a showroom floor. If you buy a secondhand crib, however, be sure the slats of the sides are no more than 2⅜ inches apart and that the mattress fits snugly to the inside edges of the crib.

Housing

A safe, healthy environment is often difficult to manage. Consider the situation as well as the lodgings themselves. Is it convenient for managing a baby? A toddler? A preschooler? Is there a place nearby for walks and for safe play? Do you have access to stores, health care, relatives, or to other caretakers if they are needed?

The following is a check list of basics you should look for in the home you provide for your baby:

- Is there reasonable privacy for a crying baby?

- Can you take the baby outdoors safely, not just as an infant but also as an exploring toddler?

- Are stores, health care, caretakers, and other needed services reasonably convenient?

- Can the home be reasonably childproofed, including the stairs, windows, storage areas, etc.?

- Is the home in good enough repair to paint, decorate, and make attractive?

- Are the home and surroundings free of bugs and rodents?

- Is the plumbing and electrical wiring reasonably new, adequate, and safe?

- Is the water supply pure and wholesome?

- Is the level of air pollution and noise pollution acceptable in the neighborhood?

- Is there a safe, reliable source of heat?

- If there are stoves or space heaters, are they safe and safely installed according to fire safety codes? Are there smoke detectors in good working order?

- Is the flooring safe and free of nails and splinters?

- Are walls, sills, and other surfaces free of lead-containing paint?

Protecting Your Child—Accident Prevention

More children die as a result of accidents, in the age group from one to four years, than from the next seven leading causes of child death combined! In addition, every year, one-third of the entire child population under age six receives some injury requiring medical attention. Two-thirds of all accidents occur in the home. And the discouraging fact of these statistics is that although other causes of child death and disability have been declining during the past decade, death and disability from accidents have remained the same.

When a baby is very young, parents have the entire responsibility to prevent accidents. As the child grows and begins to understand his environment, the responsibility becomes shared. The child must learn to take over responsibility for his own welfare. Parents must think both in terms of protecting the child and teaching him so that the responsibility for accident prevention can eventually be transferred from parent to child as the child matures. While the learning process is going on, safety rules must be absolute and applied with strict consistency. This goes for the entire family regardless of age. Remember that you and older siblings are role models for the babies of the family. You can caution a child until you are blue in the face about not running into the street, but if he sees you or an older brother or sister do it, he will, too. If you make lighting a cigarette with matches look attractive, you can bet your child will try it despite any warnings you might give against it.

Promoting child safety is a very difficult proposition. You have to allow exploration and experimentation while setting limits consistent with your child's age and the abilities she has developed. You want to teach and caution your child about danger without making her a fearful child.

As soon as a child begins understanding words, explain dangers and teach her about them. But don't expect a lot of understanding until some time between the ages of two-and-one-half and three years. Along with your teaching, you will have to physically remove your child from danger and express your disapproval of dangerous actions. Children from age one on will explore and experiment dangerously despite your warnings; they will test your limits and the limits of their own abilities until you put a stop to whatever they are doing.

But along with the *no*s, you should provide many *yes*es and as much teaching as you can manage. Praise proper actions when your toddler is playing well with safe toys. Allow harmless play even if it is messy and save the nos for more important occasions.

With ingenuity you can teach some lessons. For example, a child won't know what "It will burn you" means until he has burned himself. Make a lamp with a forty-watt bulb available to touch while you are in attendance. Warn, "It will burn you" and probably the baby will touch it anyhow.

It won't do any damage, but the baby will get the feel of being burned. Sympathize with him and tell him clearly, "Oh, it burned you!" Next time, he may understand when you tell him the same thing about a stove or radiator.

In similar ways, without hurting your child, you can teach her that pointed objects can hurt, ropes can hurt, and playground swings can hurt when they bump her. Play acting may be effective. Pretend to burn yourself on your kitchen stove. Make quite a scene about it and let your child comfort you and help "make it better." Emphasize, "Oh, I burned myself!" When your toddler has a small but painful fall, tell her how she hurt herself falling as you comfort her. You want your child to learn the sources of hurts so that she slowly comes to assume the responsibility for protecting herself. Demonstrate auto safety by using a seat belt yourself. Exaggerate looking both ways as you cross a street. Set a good example other times: don't snatch up your child and dash through traffic on a shortcut to the store if you don't want her to do the same thing another time.

Following are eight major classes of accidents and tips for their prevention. It's almost impossible to protect your child from himself and his environment all of the time, but read the frightening accident statistics at the beginning of this section once again and do the best you can.

Motor Vehicle Accidents

- Use an approved infant or child auto seat that is properly restrained. Refer to recent reports in a consumer magazine for the best restraint for your child's age (ask your librarian to direct you to consumer reports). After age four, use regular seat belts. Keep informed about the latest information on airbags, and the best location in an automobile for small children. A properly restrained child in a back seat is the safest place according to current thinking. Front-seat air bags in their current state of technology can be a threat to children. Keep yourself informed as new technologies are developed.

- Children under three must be carefully supervised in a fenced play area to keep them from running into the road.

- Older children must be educated not to play behind a parked car under any circumstances, especially in a box, a pile of leaves, or in snow.

- Educate your child in safe bike riding. Be sure the child wears a helmet.

- Forbid pursuing anything into the road or crossing a road unsupervised under age six. Street-crossing education should begin by age three and continue through early school years. Be more particular about streets with heavy traffic.

- To avoid slamming fingers or hands in the car door, play a simple game when loading children in a car: say, "Simon says hands on head!" Don't slam the door until all hands are on heads. Never close an overhead garage door until all children are well clear of it.

Drowning

- Never leave an infant untended in the bath for even a minute. Never leave a filled tub

unguarded. Supervise bathing at least to age four.

- Most child drownings in pools or other bodies of water occur in shallow water, as little as six inches!

- All children must be closely supervised when any pool or other body of water is nearby, including swamps, intermittent streams, and culverts. Children under three should be restrained when outdoors.

- Teach swimming as young as possible. Age one is not too soon if you use a qualified instructor; or learn how to teach him yourself.

- Teach water safety, not water fear, from about age two. If you are afraid of water yourself, leave the instruction to someone who respects but does not fear water. When a frightened child falls in water she may panic and drown when all she has to do is stand up.

- A child should wear a flotation device around deep water until he is a dependable swimmer; flotation devices should be worn in boats at all times.

- Learn and practice resuscitation procedures.

Burns

- Controls of cooking stoves should be out of reach of toddlers.

- Children should not be left in the kitchen unsupervised.

- Provide guards for stoves and radiators. Electric space heaters should be out of reach.

- Teach the meaning of "It will burn you." (See prefacing remarks.)

- Forbid playing with lamp and appliance cords, even when unplugged. Forbid play near the TV and other appliances.

- Use plastic plug guards in all unused outlets.

- Keep electric appliances away from the bath area.

- Learn and practice resuscitation procedures.

- Turn pot handles to the back of the stove.

- Don't use tablecloths with long skirts that can be pulled.

- Keep your child out from underfoot when you pour hot liquids.

- Always test your child's bath water.

- Have your plumber or heating repair man limit household water temperature to 125°F or less.

- Keep steam vaporizers out of reach. Don't direct the steam jet at the child. Use a cool-mist vaporizer.

- Infant skin is very sensitive to sun. Keep infants shaded, including the head. Use sunscreen lotions on older children. Limit time spent in the sun.

- Have your home safety-checked for fire hazards: faulty wiring and electrical overloads; improperly installed or vented

stoves; space heaters and irons near flammable material, etc.

- Keep matches out of reach, preferably locked up.

- Quit smoking. Most home fires are caused by smokers.

- Use flame-retardant sleepwear. Read labels. After many washings, however, fabrics lose retardant qualities.

- Never leave children unsupervised when there is an outdoor fire, such as a barbeque, leaf burning, or campfire.

Poisons

- If you move into an old house, have the paint on walls and sills analyzed for lead. Take a chip of paint from next to bare wood, not from more recent layers. Find the name of a testing laboratory in the yellow pages or ask the pediatric section of your local hospital for a referral. Also check painted secondhand cribs.

- Keep plants out of reach. Hanging plants are best but be alert for any dropped leaves or flowers on the floor.

- Know the names of your plants and label them. There are seven hundred species of plants known to cause illness or death. If your plants are labeled, you will know what to tell your doctor or the poison center if your baby eats any of them.

- Storing cleaning solutions, sprays and insecticides, automobile fluids, etc., in high, locked cabinets is best but not always possible. Second best is fitting cabinets with difficult latches. Inquire at the hardware store. Use as few storage cabinets as possible, so you won't have to childproof many. Attach a small bell to dangerous cabinets, so you will be warned to come running.

- Most poisoning occurs in the kitchen. Don't allow children in the kitchen unsupervised. Keep cleaning products on top shelves. Toilet and drain cleaners are highly alkaline and can do horrible damage to mouth parts and the esophagus.

- Don't store anything in food containers except food. Antifreeze solutions are often sweet tasting. If a dangerous solution is stored in a soda bottle, a child may think it is soda and drink it.

- Keep medicines (even vitamins) in child-proof containers.

- Attach a bell to the medicine cabinet.

- Don't leave purses or grocery bags containing medicines lying about.

- Don't pretend drugs are candy or "yummy" when giving them to children.

- Know the phone number of your area's posion information center. It's in the front of the phone book.

Falling

- Never leave an infant alone for a moment on a high surface. Even newborns can wiggle off a table with reflex movements. At three or four months, an infant will make his first rollover when you least expect it.

- Change a wiggly child on a low bed or on the floor.

- Get in the habit of pulling up the sides of a crib even if a child can't climb out. He'll soon be old enough to try.

- Once a child is thirty-six inches or can climb over raised sides, give her a bed.

- A baby must be both restrained and attended in highchairs, table seats, swings, rockers, and playground equipment.

- Playground safety should be taught from toddlerhood on.

- Inside stairs should be blocked with folding gates at both top and bottom.

- Doors leading to hallways, stairwells, and fire escapes should be locked with hooks or locks above a child's reach.

- Have sturdy screens at open windows or fit with bars that a child can't remove but which can be removed easily if the window is needed as a fire escape.

- Guard windows as above. Keep doors locked or hooked, out of reach of the child.

- Teach children to carry pointed objects down when walking with them. Running while carrying objects with the potential to cause injury should be forbidden.

Aspiration

- Because there are so many ways a child can breathe in a small object or choke on food, know your emergency procedure for choking (see Chapter 16). Balloons can be inhaled and cut off breathing when a child tries to blow it up.

- Avoid toys with small, detachable parts and pieces small enough to swallow.

- Keep the floor and furniture clear of anything that can be swallowed, such as pins, coins, jewelry, pegs, tacks.

- Avoid nuts, raisins, and fruits with pits until you are sure your baby can handle these expertly.

- Don't give chunks of food larger or tougher than your child can handle easily.

- Avoid bony fish; avoid bones of all kinds.

- Avoid foods with crumbs that can be inhaled, caraway seeds, powdered sugar, and other toppings until your child has proved he can manage these things.

- Avoid uncontrolled laughing and fooling around at mealtime.

- Avoid chewing gum.

- Pacifiers should be of one-piece construction with a mouth shield and grasping handle.

Suffocation and Strangulation

- Remove locks, doors, and lids from refrigerators, ovens, and all kinds of chests not in use. Better yet, get rid of them.

- Educate preschoolers to the danger of crawling into things.

- Destroy plastic dry cleaning bags and other large plastic bags.

- Keep trash bags locked up, out of reach.

- Don't use plastic covers on pillows or mattresses.

- Be aware that venetian blinds, both the ropes and the slats, are strangulation hazards.

- Fasten restraining straps snugly on highchairs, swings, etc. A child can slide through loose straps and get caught by the neck.

- Don't tuck in blankets around infants. Pillows are unnecessary. Infants can wiggle free of loose blankets and small pillows. Don't confuse suffocation with crib death or sudden infant death syndrome (SIDS). The cause of SIDS is still unknown.

- Crib slats should be no more than $2\frac{3}{8}$th inches apart (the width of three of your fingers).

- Mattresses and bumper pads must fit snugly—no more than an inch clearance on sides and ends. If the space is larger, fill it in with rolled sheets or towels.

- Position a crib clear of large furniture where a child can become caught in between.

- Don't leave anything tied around a baby's neck when he is sleeping or unattended, such as a bib, beads, a bandana, or a scarf.

- Do not attach toys to a crib or playpen with a string.

- Teach toddlers and preschoolers not to play games with ropes, such as cowboy, tying to a tree or post, tying to the body with rope in any way, pretend hanging, tree or mountain climbing with rope.

Accidents While Playing and Exploring

- Handguns are designed to kill people. They often kill babies and small children. Get rid of them.

- Keep rifles and shotguns locked up and out of reach—unloaded!

- Keep ammunition, arrows, knives, and fishing gear locked up and out of reach.

- Toddlers fall a lot. Remove low furniture with sharp points and edges, such as coffee tables.

- Restrict whirling and falling down games to safe areas, such as lawns, open playrooms.

- Restrict running in dangerous areas, such as pool areas, rocky ground, or where there are curbs or other obstacles.

- Teach preschoolers playground safety.

- Teach children not to run holding sharp implements, such as scissors or pencils. No running with spoons, forks, lollipops, or anything else in the mouth.

- Select toys appropriate to a child's age. Soft toys or wood toys with rounded corners (lacking points) are best for toddlers.

- Keep all tools locked up. Disconnect table saws, grinders, lathes, etc.

- Keep children away when you are operating any power equipment. This includes lawnmowers, which can throw stones with lethal velocity.

CHAPTER 16

HOW TO RECOGNIZE AND DEAL WITH MEDICAL EMERGENCIES

When emergencies occur, you must respond immediately. Medical emergencies include loss of consciousness, loss of breathing, loss of heartbeat, major trauma with or without severe bleeding, choking, poisoning, electric shock, drowning, and burns. These can all be life-threatening or can cause serious and permanent disability; they all must be dealt with quickly, often in a matter of minutes. They all require professional medical attention in a hospital setting, of course, but the steps you take at the outset to stabilize the situation and activate the emergency medical system are crucial to the outcome.

The Hospital Emergency Room or the Doctor's Office?

Once you've established a good working relationship with your doctor, it's only natural to head for his office in times of crisis. This is usually a mistake, as your doctor will probably agree. The doctor's office does not have the staff or the equipment to enhance breathing and circulation, to transfuse blood, empty the stomach of poison, deal with severe burns, or perform operations. If your child requires this kind of help, valuable time will be lost. Transport him directly to the hospital emergency room.

Your best move is to summon an emergency medical service ambulance to your home. These services all have well-equipped emergency vehicles with a staff trained in emergency resuscitation techniques. The rescue squad will radio the emergency room for instructions on what to do at the site of the emergency and en route to the hospital. In the rare event that it seems better or more expedient to do the driving yourself, try to have a companion with you to help.

Before an emergency ever occurs, know the telephone number of your local rescue squad, usually 911. Also know the location of your nearest hospital emergency room and drive there at least once to be sure you know the way.

211

Cardiopulmonary Resuscitation (CPR)

You should know how to perform cardiopulmonary resuscitation, called CPR for short. It is employed when the heart or the lungs cease to function.

In adults, heart attack is the most common cause of cardiopulmonary arrest. In infants and children, the need for CPR is usually prompted by an airway obstruction that prevents breathing (this can, in turn, lead to cardiac arrest) or because of drowning or electric shock.

CPR has two objectives: to keep the blood oxygenated by providing air to the lungs of someone who is not breathing and to keep the blood circulating by externally compressing the heart in someone whose heart is not beating. The point of both of these maneuvers is to provide oxygen for the brain. The brain gets its oxygen from the blood. If the person is not breathing in air, the blood does not get oxygen. By breathing air into the victim's mouth, a CPR rescuer can provide some oxygen artificially. But if the heart is not beating, this oxygen will not reach the brain. Simply breathing air into the lungs of a person whose heart is not beating is a futile exercise. If both functions are absent, both must be provided for the victim. Otherwise, the cells of the brain will begin to deteriorate in about five minutes, resulting in irreversible brain damage and eventually death. The entire purpose of CPR is to maintain brain function until the patient arrives at the hospital, where definitive treatment can be given.

You cannot learn CPR by reading a book. It is not a simple technique, and you can injure a person by performing it incorrectly. You must take a course sponsored by the American Heart Association, the American Red Cross, the YMCA, your local hospital, or some other organization; they have certified instructors and mechanical mannequins on which to practice. Many high schools have qualified instructors come to train their students. Then, it is best to repeat the course every year or so as a review. In times of crisis, things have a way of flying out of your head, and you may find it hard to remember a sequence of steps you learned a long time ago.

The skills you learn in CPR may save the life of a spouse or parent as well as a child. You can make no better investment of your time than to learn this technique. No first aid kit can duplicate it, and the best emergency rescue squad can get caught in traffic. The steps you take to restore breathing and heartbeat until the rescue team arrives can mean the difference between life and death.

Choking

Choking on a foreign object or a piece of food caught in the airway is not uncommon in small children. Unfortunately, it is often fatal, and needlessly so, since almost anyone can quickly learn the proper technique for dealing with this kind of airway obstruction.

If you think your child has a foreign object in the throat that is partially obstructing the airway, open her mouth and look. If you see something you can easily reach with your fingers, pull the foreign object out promptly. Don't do this, however, if there is any danger of pushing the object further down.

If you can see that something is stuck in the throat—such as a bobby pin, toothpick, or fish bone—but the child is still able to breathe, do not attempt to remove the object yourself. Take her to the hospital emergency room where it can be removed with the proper instruments. Your attempts to remove it may push it further down and possibly cause airway obstruction.

If a foreign object blocks the airway so that the child cannot breathe, take immediate action as described below. These measures, however, are not for the child whose labored breathing is due to croup or epiglottitis (see Chapter 7). If your child has been ill with a fever, has had a barking cough, and has difficulty in breathing, he should be brought to the hospital emergency room immediately. If, on the other hand, your child has been perfectly well but suddenly starts gasping for breath (especially if he has been eating finger foods or playing with small toys), he is probably choking on a foreign object that has become lodged in the airway.

How to Deal with an Infant or a Child Who Is Choking

1. *Assess the severity of the situation.* If the child can cough forcefully, or talk, even though she may be gasping for breath, leave her alone. She may be able to expel the object herself.

   The situation may get worse, however. You can tell that this is happening if her lips, nails, and skin start to turn blue; if her coughing becomes less forceful; or if she makes high-pitched, wheezing noises while inhaling. These are signs of poor air exchange and it is at this point that you should step in. The following procedure is always taught as part of a CPR course.

2. *Position the child.* Position the child so that the head is lower than the chest.

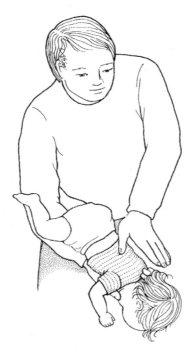

Helping a choking baby

If you are dealing with an infant, straddle her along your arm, face down, with her head cupped in your hand.

If the baby is too big for this, get down on one knee and drape the child across your other thigh, head down.

3. *Give four back blows.* Using the heel of your hand, deliver four quick, sharp blows to the back, between the shoulder blades. Use less force on an infant than you would on a child. Often this will do the trick. But if not, go to the next step.

4. *Turn the child over.* To do this with an infant, sandwich him between your two hands (always supporting the head) and flip him over. Keep him slanting downward so that the head is lower than the chest.

With a child, slip him off your thigh and roll him over onto the floor, face up.

5. *Give four chest thrusts.* If you are dealing with an infant, place two fingers of one hand on the infant's chest, midway between the nipples, and press down between one-half and one inch. Do this four times in rapid succession.

For a child, use the heel of your hand instead of two fingers, and press down between one and one-and-a-half inches.

6. *Repeat.* Repeat the sequence of back blows and chest thrusts until the obstruction is relieved.

Because food blocking the airway is one of the most common causes of choking, small children should be taught to chew their food carefully, and children under three years old should not be given hard foods like peanuts, sliced raw carrots, or tough meats because the molars needed to chew

them often have not erupted. As suggested earlier, horseplay at mealtime should not be allowed.

Poisoning

Children ingest a huge variety of harmful substances. Very few people, including most physicians, will know immediately which substances are toxic or harmless. For this reason, poison information centers exist to give emergency advice regarding suspected cases of poisoning. These centers usually have a toll-free number that is listed in the front of your telephone book along with other emergency numbers. Write the number on a self-adhering label and attach it to your telephone. Then, if your child ingests something, you will be able to contact your area's poison information center immediately for advice.

Do not depend on your intuition or on a list you may have cut out of a magazine or copied from a book to decide if something is poisonous or not. Commercial products often change their ingredients without changing the trade name. Your best source of advice on what to do is always a poison information center.

Two-year-olds are far and away the most frequent victims of accidental poisonings. Toddlers can crawl, walk, climb, unlatch safety gates, open drawers and closets, unlatch cabinets, and unscrew most lids. Children as young as four have opened the "childproof" safety caps on prescription drug containers. Not even the most vigilant parent can watch a child every minute, and a minute is all it takes for a child to get into a poison and swallow it. What parents can do is to "poison-proof" their home as much as possible by following the suggestions in Chapter 15. Following is a procedure for dealing with poisoning.

How to Deal with Poisoning

1. *End the exposure.* Empty the child's mouth of any pills, capsules, plant parts, or other substances.

2. *Identify the poison.* Save any evidence you can find that identifies the poison. This includes an open pill bottle, jar, can, or other container that held the poison, and any substance you remove from the child's mouth. Also save any vomitus that the child brings up after ingesting the poison. Bring this evidence with you to the hospital.

3. *Counteract the effects of the poison.* There are two ways to do this: by diluting the poison in the child's body, or by making him vomit it up. The method you use depends on what your child has swallowed, as explained in the following section.

Acid, Alkaline, and Petroleum Poisons

It is important that you be able to recognize a poison belonging to the acid, alkaline, or petroleum groups because these are poisons for which you do *not* induce vomiting.

Acid and alkaline poisons are corrosive poisons. These include drain cleaners; oven cleaners; bleaches; electric dishwashing granules; lye; and hydrochloric, sulfuric, nitric, and carbolic acids. They burn going down, and they will burn coming back up again. Alkaline substances found in drain and toilet cleaners are by far the most dangerous because they can do terrible damage to the mouth and esophagus.

Petroleum poisons include gasoline, kerosene, paint thinner, some garden sprays, paintbrush cleaner, lighter fluid, furniture polish, car polish, metal polish, and dry cleaning fluids. If the child vomits up these substances, they may be breathed into the lungs, where they can cause a deadly chemical pneumonia.

How to Counteract Acid, Alkaline, or Petroleum Poisons

If you have identified the poison your child has ingested as belonging to one of these three groups, you should immediately attempt to dilute the poison.

1. Try to make the child drink two glasses of milk, or if milk is not available, give water. Give the liquid slowly to avoid vomiting.

2. See that the child remains upright in a sitting or standing position to prevent the toxic substance from running back up the esophagus.

3. Rush him to the hospital.

Other Poisons

These can run the gamut from the contents of your medicine cabinet to tobacco, alcoholic beverages, mushrooms in the lawn, and plants in the house. Some seven hundred species of plants are known to cause death or illness if eaten. Among these are lily of the valley, foxglove, mountain laurel, wild buttercups, yellow jasmine, morning glory, poinsettia, mistletoe's white berries, bittersweet berries, the castor-bean plant, oleander, and plants in the rhododendron family, such as the western azalea. Apple seeds and fruit pits can also make your child ill. All of these substances should be removed from the child's stomach by inducing vomiting.

How to Induce Vomiting

The best way to induce vomiting is to administer syrup of ipecac. This is available at the drugstore and you should have it on hand in your medicine cabinet.

1. An appropriate dose of Ipecac for a child under six is one tablespoon ($\frac{1}{2}$ ounce). After giving the Ipecac, have your child drink a large glass of water, at least six ounces, and encourage her to walk around. This will make the Ipecac work faster.

2. Take your child to the nearest hospital emergency room after you have administered the Ipecac. Be sure to take along a bowl or pail for the vomitus, and a towel. The syrup of Ipecac should take effect within fifteen minutes or so.

3. If you don't have any Ipecac, you may be able to induce vomiting by gently gagging the child with your finger or with a smooth spoon handle. Much of the time, however, this does not work. You may be somewhat more successful by mixing a teaspoon or more of salt into a glass of water and having your child drink this. Water containing powdered mustard also works sometimes. Don't waste a lot of time trying different things, however. Call the emergency service or get started for the hospital and try to induce the vomiting as you go.

Do not induce vomiting in a child who is unconscious or who is having a convulsion because he may choke on the vomitus.

Burns

Young children are extremely vulnerable to burn injuries. House fires, kitchen stoves, scalding water in the shower, and chemical burns from skin contact with lye or acids are some of the many kinds of burns children can suffer.

How to Handle Your Child's Burns

1. Stop the burning process. Smother flames, don't fan them. Bring the child to the floor and roll her in a blanket or rug.

2. Try to prevent the child from inhaling flames, heat, or smoke by keeping her horizontal so that the flames do not burn toward the head. Keep the head free if you have rolled the child in a rug or blanket.

3. Cool the burn with cold water. This accomplishes four things: it relieves pain; it reduces the severity of the burn; it lessens tissue damage at the borders of the burn site, and it washes away debris or, in the case of a chemical burn, the chemical.

4. Do not apply oils, salves, butter, or ointments of any kind, but immediately take the child to the hospital. All but the most minor burns should be seen by a doctor.

Bleeding

Whenever there is bleeding, things tend to look worse than they actually are. Dabbing with a washcloth often reveals a relatively minor cut that requires just a Band-Aid.

Your child may, of course, suffer a larger cut than this. Your major objective in such cases is to stem the loss of blood until your child gets to the hospital.

How to Control Blood Loss

1. *Apply pressure.* Hold a clean cloth tightly against the bleeding area and maintain pressure on the wound.

2. *Elevate the wound.* If possible, elevate the wound so that it is above the level of the heart, thus lessening the blood flow.

In most cases, these steps will control bleeding until you can get the child to the hospital. Unless you have some expertise, do not attempt to control bleeding by finding arterial pressure points. Firm local pressure to the bleeding is usually far more effective. And don't be afraid to press hard. You won't do more damage, and if your child continues to bleed severely, he may go into shock.

If there is a knife, ski pole, or some other sharp object protruding from the wound, do not remove it. This could lead to severe, uncontrollable bleeding.

Tourniquets are rarely necessary and should be used only in extreme circumstances. A very badly mangled, or a partially or fully amputated extremity might be a situation where you would have to resort to a tourniquet.

How and When to Devise a Tourniquet

1. You will need a piece of cloth at least the size of a handkerchief. Don't use a piece of rope, wash line, or shoelace. A neck tie, a handkerchief, or a shirt sleeve are all much better choices.

2. Tie your cloth around the extremity, above the wound (toward the body).

3. Insert a sturdy stick about five inches long under the cloth. A dull table knife, a wooden cooking spoon, or even a hair brush with a long handle are all adequate substitutes. Then, twist the stick around to tighten the tourniquet until the bleeding stops.

4. Tie the stick to the tourniquet to prevent it from untwisting until you get the child to the hospital. Once the tourniquet is tightened, do not release it.

Remember, local pressure will control most bleeding. Use a tourniquet only as a last resort in the most dire emergencies.

Chest Wounds

If your child receives a chest wound and you can hear air sucking in and out of the hole, seal this hole as rapidly as possible. Put your hand over the hole when the child exhales to prevent new air being sucked in the next time the child takes a breath. A piece of plastic wrap covered with several layers of clean cloth is even better, but don't waste time looking for it. Just cover the hole immediately and keep it covered. A chest wound that is sucking air probably means that one lung is at least partially collapsed already. Time is extremely important.

If there seems to be several broken ribs and the chest has an abnormal or bulging shape in one area, support this area with your hands or with a firm pillow to prevent the bulge and keep the chest in its normal shape.

Shock

The most serious consequence of bleeding is shock. Shock (not to be confused with electric shock) is a state of circulatory collapse—that is to say, the blood is not circulating throughout the body as forcefully as it should be. If your child has lost a lot of blood, there may not be enough left to provide adequate circulation. But shock can result from other kinds of trauma besides blood loss. A child can go into shock as a result of major injury, extensive burns, poisoning, dehydration, or a severe allergic reaction to medicine or an insect sting.

It is vital to be able to recognize the signs of shock, since it is one of the direst of medical emergencies. Without treatment, shock leads quickly to coma and death.

The symptoms of shock include pallor; a cold, clammy skin; a bluish tinge to lips, nails, ear lobes, and fingertips; and rapid, shallow breathing. A child in shock may shiver and complain of being cold and thirsty. Initial feelings of anxiety will give way to apathy and disinterest.

How to Treat Shock

1. To treat shock, wrap your child in a warm blanket.

2. Keep the head lower than the rest of the body by placing pillows under the buttocks and legs.

3. Refuse requests for water; the danger is too great that the child will vomit and inhale it.

4. Get the child to the hospital in the quickest way possible—preferably by ambulance.

Back and Neck Injuries

If there has been a back or neck injury, don't move the child at all—simply call the rescue squad. If one of the neck or back vertebrae has been broken or displaced, there is a strong possibility of a spinal cord injury. You may make this substantially or even permanently worse by trying to move the child. The rescue squad will have neck collars and back-immobilizing boards for moving people with neck or back injuries.

If you must move a child because she is in the water or in the presence of fire or possible explosion, move her with as little neck and back motion as possible. Don't let the head fall backward, forward, or to either side. If possible, slide a board—such as a piece of plywood, a leaf from a table, a surfboard, toboggan, or even a small area rug—underneath her and drag her out. But continue to support the head and neck without moving them.

Drowning

Knowledge of cardiopulmonary resuscitation (CPR) is crucial here. Positioning the head, clearing the airway, breathing air into the lungs and, if necessary, performing external heart massage are beyond the capabilities of a person with no training. You have to know what you're doing. Don't put it off—learn CPR!

A few reminders for those of you who do know CPR: resuscitation attempts should begin immediately for drowning victims. The rescuer should begin mouth-to-mouth resuscitation when he reaches shallow water and continue on land. Vomiting is common in drowning because the stomach is filled with water. If vomiting occurs, turn the child face down to keep the water from entering the lungs. The lungs of drowning victims, by the way, are usually free of water because the larynx goes into spasm.

As soon as possible after rescue, call the rescue squad and have the child transported to the nearest hospital emergency room. Continue resuscitation until help arrives. Children have been known to survive long periods of immersion in water, particularly if the victim has been in very cold water. Some children who have fallen through the ice on frozen rivers have been successfully resuscitated with no apparent damage after being in the water for as long as forty-five minutes.

Electric Shock and Electrocution

Electric shocks and electrocution happen when a child comes in contact with a fallen high tension wire, when she sticks a metal object into a wall outlet, when she puts a finger in an electric light socket, or when she touches a bare wire, especially when she is standing in bare feet on a wet floor. You must immediately remove the electric source from the child if she is still in contact with it. Do this using a nonconducting item such as a wooden stick or chair. If the child has stopped breathing, you will have to breathe for her; if her heart has stopped beating, you will have to proceed with external heart massage until the emergency rescue squad arrives. Once again, knowledge of CPR is essential.

Sudden Infant Death Syndrome (SIDS)

One of the most tragic and devastating occurrences is the sudden and unexpected death of a baby. Sudden Infant Death Syndrome (SIDS) characteristically strikes during sleep. Typically, the infant has been entirely healthy or may have had a very mild upper respiratory infection. Death comes silently and the parents usually discover it when they go in to check the baby before they retire, or they get up in the morning to find the baby dead.

Parents who experience this tragedy must understand that there is nothing they could have done to prevent it. The baby did not suffocate because of the way you positioned him in the crib; he did not "hurt himself" in the crib; he did not die of neglect, nor did he cry out to an unhearing caretaker. The death was silent, sudden, and unpredictable.

SIDS occurs most frequently between the ages of two and four months, rarely before two weeks or beyond six months of age. It is the largest single cause of infant death after the neonatal period.

Though theories abound, no definitive cause of SIDS has been verified. It has been observed that infants who experience an episode of otherwise unexplained, nonfatal respiratory arrest (cessation of breathing) have a higher risk of dying of SIDS. Such an episode might last for twenty seconds or so before the infant begins breathing again—often when the parent shakes him and calls his name. Home monitoring machines have been devised that will sound an alarm should the baby stop breathing. A high-risk infant can be hooked up to such a machine every night until the doctor feels the baby is no longer at risk. If you think your infant has suffered an episode of respiratory arrest, do not delay in telling your doctor about it.

It has also been observed that there is a lower incidence of SIDS among infants who are positioned on their back or on their side in the crib which, at this writing, has caused doctors to recommend putting a very young baby to bed this way. But then, babies who do a lot of spitting up are at risk of breathing in vomit if they are on their back.

Parents who have lost a baby to SIDS should contact the social services department of their hospital to find a support group that helps families in this situation.

Unconsciousness

If your child is unconscious or cannot be fully aroused with substantial stimulation, get her to the emergency room immediately. Don't use CPR if she is breathing normally and has a normal heartbeat.

If your child is a known diabetic and seems on the verge of unconsciousness, try and get her to drink some heavily sweetened orange juice, sugar water, or other liquid into which you have mixed a large amount of sugar. If she is unconscious or can't swallow, don't attempt to force her to drink.

Convulsions

Convulsions are among the most frightening of medical events. (Refer to Chapter 10 for a description of a grand mal or febrile convulsion.) A first epileptic seizure can occur at any age. Once a convulsion has started, there is nothing you can do to stop it. Most convulsions last considerably less than five minutes; some, less than a minute. All you can do is try to prevent your child from injuring himself during the convulsion.

How to Deal with a Convulsion

1. Do not attempt to move the child during the seizure. Simply move away furniture or other objects he might strike with an arm or leg during the uncontrolled, jerking movements. If he is in a dangerous place, move him as short a distance as possible.

2. Loosen any tight clothing.

3. If he begins to vomit or the secretions in his mouth become heavy, turn him to one side or onto his stomach.

4. Do not put anything in his mouth to try to prevent him from biting his tongue. He may have already done this with the first few violent jerks and putting something in his mouth is likely to cause further injury.

5. Do not try to restrain him or hold the jerking limbs. You will not succeed and may cause some damage.

6. Do not attempt mouth-to-mouth resuscitation. It is perfectly normal for a child to stop breathing momentarily during a seizure. He will start breathing again on his own.

7. When the seizure is over, your child will want to sleep. If this is the first seizure he has had, call your doctor and then take him to the nearest hospital emergency room. If he is a known epileptic and is being treated, this is not necessary. Simply keep him comfortable at home and let him rest until he awakens.

Children with febrile convulsions, which are brought on by a rapid rise in body temperature, should be cooled as rapidly as possible. Remove the clothing and sponge the child with tepid water that is warm enough so that the child does not shiver violently, but cool enough to have some significant cooling effect. When the seizure has stopped and you have achieved some degree of cooling, call your doctor and take your child to the hospital. If he is able to take it, give your child acetaminophen.

CHAPTER 17

HOW TO CREATE A MEDICAL HISTORY AND HEALTH RECORD FOR YOUR BABY

Parents can create a unique and valuable gift for their baby that no one else can duplicate—a complete and documented medical history and personal health record. It's a gift that follows your baby throughout life, contributing to health decisions that will be made far into the future.

Why You Should Keep a Health Record for Your Baby

Babies grow up quickly, accomplishing more growth in the first five years than at any other period of their lives. Many events are compressed into a short space of time and you can't possibly remember them all. The weight gains and new skills acquired seem momentous at the time they are happening, but they are continually being replaced by new and equally momentous events, and the earlier ones are forgotten.

Then there are simple things like childhood diseases and immunizations that have significance

for years to come. If your child is injured five years from now, will you remember if he was inoculated against tetanus? What about rubella, pertussis, and hepatitis? You may even have forgotten what these things are much less whether your child has been protected against them. Will you remember if your baby had a strep infection at age three that may have important implications now that she's ten?

Some events have long-range effects that cannot even be guessed at, when they happen. In the mid-1950s, for example, the hormone DES was routinely prescribed for pregnant mothers with a history of miscarriages. These mothers unwittingly passed on a ticking time bomb to their daughters in the form of an increased risk of genital cancer when they reached childbearing age. Monitoring these daughters at risk was crucial to their health. But how to identify them? Most mothers would be hard pressed to recall a drug taken for a short while some twenty or thirty years ago. New drugs appear continually, and while they are deemed safe on the basis of tests on thousands of people, long-term

221

effects are often unknown. This is the kind of information you are asked to record in the prenatal section of your baby's health history.

What a Medical History Is

A medical history is a résumé of everything medically significant throughout your baby's life, including facts about health as well as details of illnesses. Among the many items contained in your child's medical history are these:

- Vital signs—normal body temperature, pulse rate, respiratory rate, blood pressure, and how these change as your child grows

- Growth statistics—height, weight, and other important measurements

- Developmental records—your baby's acquisition of new skills and whether she does so in a timely fashion

- Immunization records

- Allergies and other chronic illnesses and their treatments

- Medication records

- Accidents, injuries, and operations

- Family history

- Doctor and dentist visits and treatments

- Family history

Are Parents Qualified to Create and Keep a Medical History?

No one is in a better position to keep a baby's medical history than you are. Doctors see the baby when she is sick, or during routine visits that become less and less frequent as the baby gets older. You often see different doctors in group practices, on visits to specialists, or in the emergency room. When you move to a new home or change doctors, the medical records don't always follow. You see your child every day and can tell at a glance if she is "not herself lately" or if subtle changes are occurring that should be investigated.

Finally, only a parent can set down details of a child's ancestry—a history of heart ailments and other diseases that tend to have familial influences, or known genetic factors that may become important later in a child's life.

How to Get Started

The whole project may seem daunting at first, but it need be no more complicated than starting a file folder with your child's name on it. A large loose-leaf binder with lots of pocket pages works well, too. (And while you're at it, starting a record for each member of the family is also an excellent idea.) If your home is computerized and you are conscientious about keeping computer files, this is another way to begin. The important thing is that it be easy for you to do and easily accessible.

If you start while your child is still a baby, you don't have to range back over a number of years to fill in information. A little digging and memory searching may be necessary for older members of the family. All the questions you need to answer can be found in the following pages. Start by completing the questions about your baby's family background and prenatal history under "Compiling a History and Gathering Records" later in this chapter. Call the doctor's office to fill in any gaps. The office assistant can answer most of your questions. Then keep things up to date as events unfold and visits to the doctor occur. It's an extra effort to catch up once you've fallen behind. If you are pressed for time, just drop a note in the file or in a pocket of your looseleaf record and fill in the details later.

Make It a Family Project

Keeping a medical history and health record can be a fascinating and educational family project. Most of the tests you have read about in this book are easy and fun to do, and they educate family members about their bodies and how they work. As you make entries you will have an opportunity to discuss good health habits, and you may have a chance to expose and discuss a child's hidden fears that may not come to light otherwise.

As your child grows, he can assume some of the responsibility for tracking his own health— weighing himself, learning how to take blood pressure, learning the parts of the body and the names of teeth, and so on. Let him know that one day these records will be his and it will be part of his family history when he has children of his own.

Compiling a History and Gathering Records

Getting Started

1. Start a page with the basics: name; date of birth; names of mother, father, grandparents, brothers, and sisters.

2. Name and address of the hospital or other place where baby was born.

3. Names of doctors, midwives, and nurses in attendance at the birth.

4. Name, address, and phone number of your pediatrician.

5. Make a note of emergency phone numbers.

Prenatal History

1. Enter father and mother's blood group and Rh factor. You can get this by calling your doctor's office. When you have prenatal blood tests, be sure to ask for the results and have them explained if necessary.

2. List all drugs taken during pregnancy, with the strength of each and the frequency of use.

3. Record the results of all prenatal tests performed: x-rays, ultrasound, amniocentesis, and so on. Ask your doctor to explain the results and significance of any tests you have done.

4. Record any problems you had during pregnancy and what was done about them.

Family History

1. Describe the following things about the parents, siblings, and grandparents and update this record as important changes occur.

   - Age, ethnic origin, and place of birth
   - Age of death if not living and cause of death
   - Chronic illnesses of each family member
   - Present health of each family member

2. If there seems to be some familial trait that is remarkable, describe who in the family has it among the baby's aunts and uncles as well as the parents and grandparents.

Records of the Newborn

The Newborn

1. Record the Apgar score (see Chapter 1)

2. Weight and length

3. Head circumference

4. Weight/length ratio (see Chapter 14)

5. Your observations and thoughts about your new baby

Vital Signs

These are things that you update regularly as your baby grows. Record the date and age of your child with each entry.

1. Normal body temperature and site where taken (mouth, rectum, under the arm)

2. Pulse

3. Respiratory rate

4. Blood pressure

Immunization Record

Record all immunization procedures as they happen. When your doctor tells you that booster shots will be required for a certain immunization, leave room and make a record of the time your baby should receive them.

1. DTP (diphtheria, tetanus, and pertussis [whooping cough]). Usually started at 2 months with follow-ups at 4 months, 6 months, 12 to 18 months, and between ages 4 and 6 years. Consult your doctor for a schedule and keep track. Boosters for tetanus are a good idea at age 11 and every ten years afterward.

2. Polio vaccine. Usually recommended at 2 months, 4 months, 12 to 18 months, and between ages 4 to 6 years.

3. MMR (measles, mumps, rubella [German measles]). These are usually given between 12 and 15 months with a follow-up between ages 4 to 6 years; sometimes later. Consult your doctor and keep track.

4. Vaccine against hepatitis B is usually given at birth, 2 to 4 months, 6 to 18 months, and again at age 11 or 12 years.

5. At the present time, most doctors recommend immunization against chicken pox. Keep abreast of current trends and discuss them with your doctor. If a child is age 12, has not had chicken pox, and has not been immunized, discuss immunization with your doctor.

6. Hib (Haemophilus influenza b). This is a vaccine usually given starting at two months of age. Your doctor will advise you about necessary boosters. This will help protect your child against certain bacteria that may cause a serious condition called epiglottitis (described in Chapters 3 and 7) and one form of meningitis.

Growth and Development Records

Track your child's physical growth using the National Center for Health Statistics growth charts in Chapter 14. Record the dates of developmental milestones that are explained in that chapter.

If your baby doesn't follow an established growth curve or falls considerably behind in the developmental milestones, bring it to the attention of your doctor.

Growth

1. Head circumference. Track from birth to 30 or 36 months.

2. Length. Track from birth to 36 months.

3. Stature (height). Track from ages 3 to 18 years.

4. Weight. Track from birth to 36 months.

5. Weight versus length. Track from birth to 36 months.

6. Weight versus height. Track from age 3 to 18 years.

Gross Motor Milestones

1. Head control

   - Holds head upright when held in sitting position. Average 2 to 4 months.

   - No head lag when pulled to a sitting position. Average 3 to 5 months

2. Rolling over

   - Rolls front to back. Average 3 to 6 months.

   - Rolls back to front. Average 4 to 7 months.

3. Sitting

   - Sits with some support. Average 6 to 7 months.

   - Sits straight without support. Average 8 to 10 months.

4. Walking

   - Attempts at stepping. Average 10 to 12 months.

   - Independent stepping. Average 11 to 14 months.

Fine Motor Milestones

1. Whole-hand grasp on an object (besides your finger). Average 3 months.

2. Grasps an object with thumb and forefinger. Average 8 to 9 months.

3. Builds a two-block tower. Average 12 to 15 months.

4. Holds a crayon and scribbles. Average 12 to 18 months.

Language Milestones

1. Babbling throat sounds. Average 4 weeks.

2. Babbling single sounds. Average 2 to 3 months.

3. Babbling with variations of tone and pitch. Average 6 months.

4. First words. Average 9 to 12 months.

5. Pointing to a named body part and saying it. Average 18 to 24 months.

6. Combining two words. Average 20 months.

7. Rudimentary conversation. Average 24 months.

Social Milestones

1. Social smile. Average 1 to 3 months.

2. First games (peekaboo, counting toes, etc.). Average 6 to 8 months.

3. Parallel play (with another child present). Average 18 to 24 months.

4. Wants to do everything herself. *No* is a favorite word. Average 24 to 30 months.

Keeping a Health Diary

When you have been with the same doctor for a number of years, you notice that he or she brings a rather thick folder into the examination room when you visit for one reason or another. This, of course, is a record of the ailments you have complained about over the years and the treatments prescribed for them. You should have the same sort of information in your child's health history.

Every time you and your child visit the doctor, make a note of why you went there, what the diagnosis was, and what treatment was prescribed. This should be a single page in your looseleaf book or file folder. Keep these chronologically. Then you should add information that the doctor can't, such as the following:

- How did you suspect your child needed to see the doctor?

- How long did the illness last?

- How did your child respond to the treatment?

- If the condition is a chronic one, what seems to work best and what does not seem to work?

- Have you discovered treatments yourself that seem beneficial that you want to ask the doctor about on your next visit?

This is all information that becomes useful if a condition recurs years later or if something else develops that may be related to it. It is also information that won't be easily available if you change doctors for one reason or another—which is quite a common occurrence today. If the condition is a chronic one—such as asthma, diabetes, or a growth disorder—you will want to keep a special file for this in order to keep track of what has been done and what progress is being made. Operations and other lengthy or serious procedures should also have their separate files or pages.

Eye and Teeth Records

Two body systems that require regular visits to specialists throughout a child's life are the eyes and the teeth, so records of visits to the eye doctor and the dentist should each have a separate section in your child's medical file.

Dental Records

1. Ask your dentist for a copy of a tooth chart like the one in Chapter 8. Every dentist has pads of these that she uses to record the condition of your child's teeth and what she has done on each visit.

2. Name each tooth that was worked on and describe what was done.

3. Make a record of any follow-up home treatment that was recommended.

4. Dentists often make you aware of work that might need to be done in the future. Make a record of this.

Eye Examination Records

1. Record your child's visual acuity as determined by eye-chart testing: 20/20, 20/30, etc.

2. If your child is given a prescription for eyeglasses, keep a record of the prescription.

Record and date new prescriptions as they are changed.

3. If your child wears eyeglasses, keep a record of his visual acuity with and without the glasses.

4. If your child's eyes are treated for disease or muscle imbalance, keep careful records of each visit to the doctor, treatments prescribed, and how your child's condition responded to the treatment.

Parenting and Emotional Problems

1. Record anything you consider significant in your child's behavior—the good as well as the bad.

2. If there is some continuing problem that requires visits to a psychiatrist, psychologist, or other counselor, keep a separate file to record visits, treatments, and progress.